Acute and Critical Care in Adult Nursing

Desiree Tait, David Barton,
Jane James and Catherine Williams

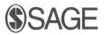

Los Angeles | London | New Delhi
Singapore | Washington DC

www.learningmatters.co.uk

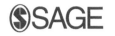

Los Angeles | London | New Delhi
Singapore | Washington DC

www.learningmatters.co.uk

Learning Matters
An imprint of SAGE Publications Ltd
1 Oliver's Yard
55 City Road
London EC1Y 1SP

SAGE Publications Inc.
2455 Teller Road
Thousand Oaks, California 91320

SAGE Publications India Pvt Ltd
B 1/I 1 Mohan Cooperative Industrial Area
Mathura Road
New Delhi 110 044

SAGE Publications Asia-Pacific Pte Ltd
3 Church Street
#10–04 Samsung   ub
Singapore 049483

Editor: Becky Taylor
Development editor: Caroline Sheldrick
Production controller: Chris Marke
Project management: Diana Chambers
Marketing manager: Tamara Navaratnam
Cover design: Toucan Design
Typeset by: Kelly Winter
Printed by: MPG Books Group, Bodmin, Cornwall

Library of Congress Control Number: 2012933560

British Library Cataloguing in Publication data

A catalogue record for this book is available from
the British Library

ISBN 978 0 85725 645 4 (paper)
ISBN 978 0 85725 842 7 (cloth)

FSC

Contents

About the authors

Desi Tait DNSc, MSc Nursing, DNE, DN, RGN is Lecturer and Team Coordinator for critical care nursing in the Department of Nursing, College of Human and Health Sciences in Swansea University. Desi has 30 years' experience in the practice, theory and education of adult acute and critical care nursing and facilitates critical care education at both undergraduate and post-graduate levels. She has a particular interest in the use of blended learning strategies in critical care undergraduate education and is involved in developing and evaluating innovative ways to facilitate student learning by adopting a practice-based approach to education. Desi completed her doctorate in the study of nurses' experience of recognising and managing clinical deterioration in patients in hospital in 2009, and this continues to be an area of clinical interest.

David Barton PhD, MPhil, BEd, RNT, DipN, RGN is Academic Lead in the Department of Nursing, College of Human and Health Science in Swansea University. David qualified as an RGN at King's College Hospital in London in 1983 and subsequently specialised in critical care nursing. Moving to Wales in 1985, he worked in Intensive Care in both Carmarthen and Swansea before becoming a Nurse Lecturer at the University of Wales Swansea in 1989. Throughout his career as a lecturer he has maintained his clinical practice, working regularly in Intensive Care. David's academic and scholarly interests have focused particularly on advanced clinical nursing, and he has worked to develop nursing networks in Wales and the UK. He is the Chair of the Association of Advanced Nursing Practice Educators (AANPE) that represents the interests of 47 universities in the UK engaged in Advanced Practice Education. David is actively involved with the Modernising Careers agenda at a strategic level both in Wales and nationally. He has also published in journals and textbooks. Recently David has taken the lead in managing the Department of Nursing at Swansea University, promoting the educational and research agenda students at pre- and post-registration level, and from undergraduate to doctoral level.

Jane James MSc Nursing, PGCE, RNT, RGN is Nurse Tutor at the College of Human and Health Sciences. She began her nursing career over 30 years ago in West Yorkshire where she specialised in Intensive Care Nursing with an interest in Neurosurgical Nursing. Later, moving to Wales, she gained experience in Acute Medical Nursing before moving into nurse education. She teaches clinical skills on the undergraduate nursing programme and has a specific interest in the use of simulation to aid learning. Jane also has a role in the selection and admission of undergraduate nursing students to the university and takes great pleasure in seeing these students progress to graduation and qualification.

Catherine Williams MSc Nursing, BSc (Hons) Nursing, PGCE, RNT, RN is Nurse Tutor/Coordinator for clinical skills education and Common Foundation Programme Manager at the College of Health and Human Sciences. She began her nursing career in 1996 and through the following years she has gained a vast array of knowledge and skills in critical care and in burns and reconstructive surgery. Catherine's role demonstrates her commitment to teaching and coordinating clinical skills education for an undergraduate pre-registration nursing programme that reflect her research interest, and she maintains her high level of clinical skills by retaining strong links with clinical practice.

Acknowledgements

The authors and publishers wish to thank the following for permission to reproduce copyright material.

The American College of Chest Physicians for Figure 7.1: The relationships between infection: SIRS, sepsis and severe sepsis, from R C Bone, R A Balk, F B Cerra, R P Dellinger, A M Fein, W A Knaus, R M Schein and W J Sibbald *Definitions for sepsis and organ failure and guidelines for the use of innovative therapies in sepsis.* The ACCP/SCCM Consensus Conference Committee.

Ron Daniels for Figure 7.2: Sepsis and severe sepsis screening, a multidisciplinary assessment, from Ron Daniels, *Surviving Sepsis Campaign* (2011).

The Intensive Care Society for Table 1.1: Defining levels of critical care, from ICS, *Levels of critical care for adult patients* (2009), Intensive Care Society, Churchill House, 35 Red Lion Square, London WC1R 4SG.

National Institute for Health and Clinical Excellence (NICE) for material in Table 1.2; from the NICE NGSO (NICE, 2007a).

Foreword

Nurses working in any setting – acute, clinical or community – will need to be prepared to recognise and respond to episodes of acute illness and apply the principles of critical care nursing in emergencies. The authors of this text have a wealth of experience that they bring together to provide second- and third-year student nurses, and post-qualifying nurses who wish to keep current, the essential ingredients to be prepared for such episodes. Acute care is characterised by its rapid, severe onset and is often short-lived. Accurate assessment is vital and nurses need to be confident in their understanding of what is happening and what to do in these circumstances. This text provides expert instruction to undertake rapid clinical assessments and use effective decision-making skills in these situations.

As well direction on assessment and accurate nursing responses, the authors (Desi Tait, Thomas Barton, Jane James and Catherine Williams) take you through the related pathophysiology of conditions and the all-important rationales underpinning the management of critically ill patients. All too often an acute episode will also involve the family and friends of a patient, which is why this text also takes this dimension of care into account in the nursing care plans. The importance of collaborative working is also not overlooked, as an understanding of professional responsibilities, within effective multiprofessional teams, is crucial in these scenarios. Considering these wider features of acute and critical care deepens your knowledge and understanding, which in turn develops your confidence and competence.

The book contains a wealth of information on specific conditions such as respiratory support, chest pain, dealing with shock and sepsis, confusion and delirium, and physical and psychological trauma. These are dealt with in specific chapters and are explained clearly, with scenarios to enable you to integrate the information in real-life situations. They are helpfully structured into chapters that you can dip into when you need specific information on managing a critically ill person. The final chapter gives you a five-point plan to maintain your knowledge and skills, ensuring you continue in your professional life as a highly competent and skilful nurse. In each chapter the relevant NMC Standards of Proficiency and NMC essential skills are stated, and are a feature of the *Transforming Nursing Practice* series.

This is a very welcome addition to the *Transforming Nursing Practice* series and I am sure will become essential reading for all nursing students.

Shirley Bach
Series Editor

Introduction

In the last ten years there has been a strong emphasis in health care on the importance of undertaking rapid assessment and management of acutely ill patients who show signs of clinical deterioration (National Patient Safety Agency, 2007b). This has led to the development and use of guidelines and policies that promote a structured process for risk assessment, monitoring and fast tracking of clinical information to optimise patient outcome (NICE, 2007a).

Patients become critically ill in any clinical or home setting and prompt management of their condition can reduce the risk of patient morbidity and mortality. The Nursing and Midwifery Council (NMC) has highlighted the recognition of patients' clinical deterioration and the management of unstable and critically ill patients as key skills in the Standards for Pre-registration Nursing Education (NMC, 2010). The general aim of this book is to provide you with the knowledge and professional guidance that you will need to assist you in developing the clinical knowledge, skills and self-confidence required to care for patients who are unstable, deteriorating or critically ill.

Each chapter focuses on the development of key clinical assessment and decision-making skills that you will need in the second and third year of undergraduate study in nursing and following qualification. The chapters include the use of patient scenarios to illustrate the clinical application of the knowledge and skills discussed. Issues related to the professional responsibilities of care are explored and applied in each chapter. They include: assessment, recognition and diagnosis of care; related pathophysiology and rationale for the assessment and diagnostic skills required; patient and family-focused care and collaborative working. Quick reference guides are used throughout to assist you when you practise the clinical decision-making activities and, where appropriate, you will be asked to reflect on your experiences in practice. Feedback on the activities is found at the end of each chapter. The core element of each chapter is to assist you in the development of skills in rapid assessment and response to clinical deterioration using 'Look: Listen: Feel: Measure/monitor: Respond'.

In Chapter 1 you are given an overview of the knowledge and skills required to assess, recognise and respond to acute and critical illness. The chapter introduces you to the levels of dependency for acute and critically ill patients as well as providing quick guides for rapid assessment and response to changes in the patient's condition. The quick reference guides can be applied to all subsequent chapters, giving you opportunities to rehearse the process, and apply and refine your skills.

In Chapter 2 you are introduced to the breathless patient and are guided through the care of patients with type I and type II respiratory failure. Patient conditions such as pneumonia, chronic obstructive pulmonary disease and asthma are discussed and you are given the opportunity to practise the diagnosis of patient conditions.

Chapter 3 builds on the content presented in Chapter 2 and explores the assessment and management of patients who need advanced respiratory support. The chapter focuses on patients in acute and critical care settings and also refers to situations when patients in the community may need to use advanced technology to support their respiratory function. A key assessment skill addressed in this section is the analysis of acid-base balance when assessing the respiratory needs of patients.

In Chapter 4 you are introduced to the patient with chest pain, and you will be guided through the process of chest pain assessment and management according to national guidelines.

Chapter 5 focuses on the patient in pain and explores the significance of pain in relation to the patient experience and the impact of pain on the development of critical illness. Pain assessment and management are considered in the context of holistic and collaborative care.

In Chapter 6 you will be guided through the process of assessing, recording and responding to patients in shock. There is also an opportunity for you to practise risk assessment and early recognition of patients in shock and steps to prevent the progression of shock.

Chapter 7 focuses on the risk assessment and management of patients at risk of developing sepsis and the management of patients with severe sepsis (including septic shock). You will be guided through sepsis care bundles and apply them to patient scenarios. There are opportunities to practise risk assessment for patients in acute care and in the community setting.

In Chapter 8 you are introduced to definitions of confusion and delirium. The chapter focuses on the risk assessment of patients with the potential to develop delirium and plan ways in which to prevent and/or manage patients in a state of delirium. You have an opportunity to reflect on patients you have nursed and an opportunity to risk assess patients for evidence of confusion.

Chapter 9 focuses on explaining the causes and management of the unconscious patient. The focus is on prioritising care and reducing the risks of side effects associated with loss of consciousness. Neurological assessment is discussed together with an evidence base for practice. Opportunities to practise neurological assessment and recognition of clinical deterioration in levels of consciousness are included.

In Chapter 10 you are introduced to the assessment and management of patients who have experienced physiological trauma. The chapter links well with Chapter 6 and includes the care of patients with soft tissue injuries including burns as well as patients with traumatic fractures.

Chapter 11 focuses on the assessment and management of patients with psychological trauma. You will be introduced to factors that positively and negatively affect patients and their families when the patient becomes critically ill. You are given the opportunity to reflect on your practice and consider how psychological well-being can impact on a patient's recovery.

Chapter 12 concludes the book and offers a summary of lessons learnt and an action plan for practice. You will be able to consider how you can develop either a career in acute and critical care and/or continue to utilise the lessons learnt in both hospital and community-based care.

There are explanations in the Glossary on page 213 for words in **bold** in the text.

Chapter 1
Assessing, recognising and responding to acute and critical illness

Desiree Tait

NMC Standards for Pre-registration Nursing Education

This chapter will address the following competencies:

Domain 3: Nursing practice and decision-making

Generic competencies:

3. All nurses must carry out comprehensive, systematic nursing assessments that take account of relevant physical, social, cultural, psychological, spiritual, genetic and environmental factors, in partnership with service users and others through interaction, observation and measurement.

Field-specific competencies:

7.1 Adult nurses must recognise the early signs of illness in people of all ages. They must make accurate assessments and start appropriate and timely management of those who are acutely ill, at risk of clinical deterioration, or require emergency care.

NMC Essential Skills Clusters

This chapter will address the following ESCs:

Cluster: Organisational aspects of care

9. People can trust the newly registered graduate nurse to treat them as partners and work with them to make a holistic and systematic assessment of their needs; to develop a personalised plan that is based on mutual understanding and respect for their individual situation promoting health and well-being, minimising risk of harm and promoting their safety at all times.

By entry to the register:

xx. Acts autonomously and appropriately when faced with sudden deterioration in people's physical, or psychological condition or emergency situations, abnormal vital signs, collapse, cardiac arrest, self-harm, extremely challenging behaviour, attempted suicide.

xxi. Measures, documents and interprets vital signs and acts autonomously and appropriately on findings.

Introduction

Scenario: Debby's story

After qualifying as a nurse my first job was in a coronary care unit. I had only been working in the unit for a week when a senior staff nurse asked me to double-check the resuscitation equipment because she felt that our new patient, who had been admitted with a three-hour history of chest pain, was likely to deteriorate and possibly have a cardiac arrest. The patient in question was pain free, had a respiratory rate, heart rate, temperature and blood pressure within the normal range and was in sinus rhythm. I thought, 'What is she on about?' Thirty minutes later the patient asked for a bottle to pass urine and as I pulled the curtains around him and walked away, he collapsed and went into ventricular fibrillation. The senior staff nurse was ready and the patient was resuscitated successfully. 'How did you know that was going to happen?' I asked. 'What did I miss? Why did I miss it?' The nurse replied that she just knew and that I would be able to do the same in a few months. I reflected back on the beginning of the shift and asked myself where I went wrong.

*   *Did I undertake a comprehensive patient assessment?*
*   *I had received handover on all the patients but I had not risk assessed each patient individually.*

*   *Did I know the patient's past and recent medical history?*
*   *Only a brief summary, I had not talked to the patient or read his notes.*

*   *Did I know and understand about the significance of the biochemical results related to this patient?*
*   *It was my first week on the unit and I didn't fully understand the significance of patients' biochemical results in the context of cardiac care.*

*   *Did I have knowledge and experience of caring for patients with similar or related problems?*
*   *I had only experienced the care of patients with chest pain while on a medical ward, and I had never experienced a medical emergency or a cardiac arrest.*

*   *Did I ask more experienced staff any questions or seek guidance?*
*   *No, I didn't want to appear foolish – after all, I was a qualified nurse!*

The more I reflected on this and similar incidents in those first few weeks, the more I realised that I had only just begun the process of becoming a competent and confident practitioner and that I still had some way to go.

What Debby's story illustrates is that assessing, risk assessing and managing care require complex skills that combine the following.

- Knowledge of bio-psychosocial systems.
- Knowledge of the patient.
- Knowledge of self.
- Relevant clinical experience.
- Observation and interpersonal skills.
- The ability to interpret patterns of illness and behaviour.
- The ability to interpret and manage care in rapidly changing situations.

The experienced nurse in Debby's story was able to demonstrate intuitive knowing. This is what Benner et al. (1999, p2) describe as *habits of thought and action* and allows the nurse to automatically have a clinical grasp of the situation, and anticipate and prevent potential problems. The development of these skills occurs over time and is always dependent on the history, knowledge and experience of the nurse (Higgs et al., 2008).

As a student you have the opportunity to observe and then practise these skills under supervision before you embrace them as a registered and accountable practitioner. While this book cannot equip you with all of these skills, it does highlight core skills and landmarks to guide you towards competent practice as well as guidance for developing your own practice.

Activity 1.1   *Reflection*

Think back to your experiences in the clinical setting.

- Can you identify a situation where you have been unable to understand how the nurse was able to know or anticipate clinical changes in a deteriorating patient?
- If you can, write down the story and look back on the incident after reading this chapter.
- Try to write down an action plan of how you might manage a similar situation in the future.

Hint: These reflective questions will help you to practise the skills of rapid assessment and management of a patient.

There is no outline answer at the end of the chapter as this activity is based on your own reflections.

Why is assessing and monitoring care important?

In 1860 Florence Nightingale recognised the significance of clinical observation and monitoring, and argued that it is a nursing responsibility to recognise and consider the cause of any change in a patient's clinical condition in order to save life and promote health. Nightingale writes (1860, p105):

> *The most important practical lesson that can be given to nurses is to teach them what to observe – how to observe – what symptoms indicate improvement – what the reverse – which are of importance – which are of none – which are the evidence of neglect – and what kind of neglect. All this is . . . an essential part, of the training of every nurse.*

Assessing and monitoring of the patient's condition has been a central role of the nurse for 150 years and yet a growing body of evidence recognises that nurses and other health care practitioners have been unable to provide safe care to a consistent standard for acutely ill patients and this has resulted in evidence of unnecessary distress and patient deaths on an international scale. A review of these findings is included in the research summary below.

Research summary: Suboptimal care

Evidence of suboptimal care can be traced back to the 1990s. In the USA Franklin and Matthew (1994) undertook a retrospective study of patient signs and symptoms before cardiac arrest and demonstrated that in 25% of the 150 cases studied there was evidence that the nurse had documented deterioration but failed to inform the medical team. They also found significant failings in the medical management of the patients. In the UK case studies of patients admitted to intensive care from the ward by McQuillan et al. (1998) and McGloin et al. (1999) found evidence of suboptimal care in 50% and 30% respectively of the cases studied. Both studies identified that nursing and medical staff had failed to recognise and/or report the urgency of the situation and that there was evidence of lack of continuity of care, poor supervision of junior staff and other organisational failings. The NPSA (National Patient Safety Agency) Report (2007b) further reinforced the concerns by publishing that out of 425 reported deaths in acute care, 64 were related to patient deterioration not being recognised or acted upon (15%). All of these research studies are based on retrospective analysis of case studies and cannot be considered to be gold standard evidence, but the nature and implications of the findings have triggered a national and international campaign to improve the recognition of and response to clinical deterioration (IHI (Institute for Health Care Improvement), 2011a; NICE, 2007a).

In the remainder of the chapter we will focus on how you can provide a safe but rapid assessment and response to patients with acute and critical illness.

Knowing and understanding the acutely ill patient

In order to know and understand the acutely ill patient you need to be able to define what acute care is and then the patient's potential for clinical deterioration. The Department of Health (2000) set out guidance for patient dependency levels, and these have subsequently been updated by the ICS (Intensive Care Society) (2009). The levels of care definitions follow a numerical pattern from 0 to 3 and are listed in Table 1.1. These levels of care have been used to assist in the risk assessment of patients as well as in the identification and justification of decisions made about the skill mix requirements for individual wards and units (NICE, 2007a; Smith, 2009). Knowing and understanding your patient can begin before you meet them and in some cases begins with the patient handover, followed by meeting and assessing the patient and ensuring continuity of patient-centred care.

Level of critical care criteria	Patient/clinical examples
Level 0 • Requires hospitalisation: needs can be met through normal ward care.	• Jennifer Jones is admitted for routine minor surgery. Her planned length of stay is two days and she will need post-operative monitoring and intravenous therapy for 24 hours during her stay.
Level 1 • Patients recently discharged from higher levels of care. • Patients in need of additional monitoring, clinical interventions, support or advice. • Patients requiring critical care outreach service support.	• Fred Jones has been discharged to your care from the high-dependency unit, where he received respiratory support and interventions for acute respiratory failure. • This includes any patient who requires a minimum of four-hourly observations with one or more of the following: • Continuous oxygen therapy for impaired respiratory function. • Fluid resuscitation, at risk of renal failure. • Intravenous or epidural pain management. • Presence of a tracheostomy, central venous catheter, chest drain. • Requiring neurological assessment. • Presence of co-morbidities such as diabetes. • This includes all patients who fulfil the medium risk category in the local patient at risk score (NICE 2007a).
Level 2 • Patients needing pre-operative optimisation in order to stabilise their condition prior to surgery. • Patients needing extended post-operative care. • Patients stepping down from level 3 to level 2 care.	• Mr Brown needs stabilisation and invasive monitoring of his cardiac and haemodynamic function prior to receiving a general anaesthetic for planned surgery. He has an arterial and central venous line. • Mary Smith was admitted to high-dependency care for 24 hours following a surgical carotid endarterectomy to remove plaque from the carotid artery. The surgery carries a risk of stroke and haemorrhage, and Mary requires hourly invasive haemodynamic monitoring and neurological assessment.

Table 1.1: Defining levels of critical care

Source: ICS, 2009.

Continued

Level of critical care criteria	Patient/clinical examples
Level 2 • Patients who are receiving single organ support/basic respiratory support/basic cardiovascular support. • Patients receiving advanced cardiovascular/renal/neurological/dermatological support.	• Harry required 14 days of **invasive ventilation** and is now being weaned from full respiratory support to spontaneous breathing. He has a tracheostomy, is confused at times and tires quickly. • Jane Morris has been admitted with sepsis and requires invasive haemodynamic support and oxygen therapy. • Paul Smith was admitted following a road traffic incident. He has sustained bilateral fractured shafts of femur and a fractured pelvis. He requires advanced cardiovascular support following emergency surgery to stabilise the fractures.
Level 3 • Patients receiving advanced respiratory support alone or support for a minimum of two organs.	• Ben Williams was transferred from an acute medical ward after showing signs of clinical deterioration. He is diagnosed with pneumonia, acute respiratory distress syndrome, severe sepsis and acute renal failure. He requires invasive ventilation, invasive haemodynamic support and renal replacement therapy.

Table 1.1: Continued

During handover

The levels of dependency allow you to risk assess, from a distance, the potential for patient deterioration; if the patient's dependency level is noted during handover, then you have already started to prioritise your patients' needs. Other factors, identified during handover and/or during the patient assessment that may influence the potential for the patient to deteriorate may be related to the following factors.

*   *Age*: increasing age in the older adult is associated with increased vulnerability to co-morbidities, infection, multiple medications.
*   *Hydration*: over- or under-hydration can increase the risk of clinical deterioration.
*   *Nutrition*: Malnutrition can prolong recovery, wound healing and increase the risk of infection.
*   *Pain*: A patient in pain is likely to have impaired mobility and increased risk of venous thrombosis, chest infection and a longer length of stay in hospital.
*   *Mobility*: Reduced mobility increases the risk of pressure ulcers, sepsis and lethargy.
*   *Mood/psychological*: Anxiety, fear and low mood can negatively impact on the speed and progress of a patient's recovery.
*   *Mental health*: Knowledge and understanding of patients' mental health problems can enhance your understanding of their ability to cope with other health problems.
*   *Learning difficulties*: Knowledge of underlying physiological disorders related to their learning difficulties can be crucial and vital to risk assessment of these patients.
*   *Co-morbidities and medication*: the presence of combined bio-psychosocial problems such as diabetes, heart disease and the patient's requirement for a hip replacement will increase the risk associated with surgery. Drugs such as prednisilone are steroids that, when prescribed, can lead to a suppressed immune response, hypertension and raised blood glucose.

Recognising the significance of these factors in patients will alert you to the potential for deterioration and can help to prevent deterioration – rather than waiting and responding to the deteriorating patient, as illustrated in the next scenario.

Scenario: Mrs Brown

During handover you learn that Mrs Brown (81 years) has been admitted with sepsis and pain on passing urine. She also has diabetes (type II) and a history of transient ischaemic attacks. Her blood glucose levels are >10mmols/L, P: 94, R: 20, BP 148/90. Without seeing this patient you should already be alerted to potential problems related to the risk of severe sepsis, a cardiovascular event and raised blood glucose. You can prioritise this patient as level 1 dependency, at risk of deterioration, and needing immediate risk assessment.

Meeting and assessing the patient

This should always begin with a rapid assessment of your patient's safety (illustrated in Table 1.2). If you are concerned, complete the rapid assessment and report your concerns without delay (NICE, 2007a; NPSA, 2007a). The difference between a routine assessment and a rapid assessment of a patient's condition is the ability to anticipate, recognise and respond in a timely manner to any aspect of concern you have for the patient's condition. The National Institute for Health and Clinical Excellence (NICE, 2007a) recommends that in these circumstances you should initiate and perform the admissions, recognition and response bundles and monitor the patients' conditions illustrated in Table 1.2.

Central to the use of these bundles is the integration of the physiological track and trigger score, and the use of emergency outreach teams for the provision of patient and staff support. The track and trigger score, also known as an early warning score (EWS) and patient at risk score (PAR) have been recommended by NICE (2007a) as a tool for recognising the early signs of clinical deterioration in level 0 and level 1 patients. In 2012 there are plans for a national early warning score (NEWS) to standardise risk assessment across the UK (RCP, 2012). It has been recommended by NICE that adding a numerical score and tracking the changes in the patient's

Bundle of care	Bundle purpose	Interventions
Admission bundle: multidisciplinary	To achieve a baseline of patient data within two hours of admission, collected and communicated to the medical team.	1. Minimum data to collect on admission to your practice area: T, P, R, BP, level of consciousness (LOC), oxygen saturation (SaO_2). 2. Document a clear monitoring plan including the type and frequency of observations to be undertaken. 3. Ensure that all members of the multidisciplinary team know and agree the monitoring plan.
Recognition bundle	Early identification and risk assessment of the deteriorating patient.	1. Monitor physiological signs at least 12 hourly for all patients. 2. Record track and trigger score. 3. Perform risk assessment according to the assessment and trigger score. 4. Consider the possibility of sepsis/severe sepsis. 5. Communicate the information to the medical team.
Response bundle	Optimal and timely treatment of the at-risk patient.	1. If there is clinical concern. 2. If the trigger score is in the low-risk range, increase the frequency of the observations. 3. If the trigger score is in the medium-risk range, contact the patient's medical team urgently and/or the critical care outreach team. 4. If the trigger score is in the high-risk ranges (excluding cardiac arrest), contact the critical care outreach team urgently. 5. In all cases communicate and document communication using the SBAR (situation, background, assessment, recommendation) tool.

Table 1.2: Rapid response to acute illness: admission, recognition and response bundles

Source: NICE, 2007a; NHS Wales, 2010.

condition provides objective evidence of deterioration and justifies calling the rapid response team for support. However, a systematic review of the effectiveness of physiological track and trigger tools by Gao et al. (2007) concluded that the validity, reliability and sensitivity of the tools in use were poor when used as a single indicator for evidence of deterioration.

Clinically effective detection and management of clinical deterioration therefore begins with nurses being alerted to or recognising signs of clinical deterioration and using a systematic, comprehensive and holistic approach to managing care.

When meeting and assessing the patient, it is important not to make assumptions about your patient's bio-psychosocial and spiritual needs until you have verified this with the patient and the health care team. Has your patient made a choice about resuscitation? Does your patient have a living will? The provision of patient-centred care should take into account patients' individual needs and wishes where possible. You should be encouraging patients to make informed decisions about their care, and this includes advanced care planning for decisions about cardiopulmonary resuscitation when it is appropriate to do so, for example in the patient case study below (BMA, Resuscitation Council (UK) and RCN, 2007).

Case study: Tom Jones

*Tom is 79 years old and has a 20-year history of chronic respiratory disease. For the last ten years he has been admitted to level 2 and/or 3 care for management of acute exacerbations of his chronic respiratory problem during the winter months. Last year he was in hospital for a period of 12 weeks. Tom has made it clear to his family and the nursing team that he doesn't want to go through 'that torture' again. He has expressly wished that he does not want to be '**intubated** and put on a **ventilator**'. A collaborative team meeting with Tom and his family resulted in clear documented guidelines for active treatment of his chest infection with a ceiling of treatment noted: 'He will receive active and full support for his condition excluding invasive respiratory support of any kind and cardiopulmonary resuscitation.' The documentation was agreed and signed, with review dates and criteria agreed with the patient and family.*

Knowledge of your patient will enable you to make informed decisions about your patient's progress. Where possible, plan for continuity of care using a collaborative team approach to organising patient-centred care with clear lines of responsibility and continuity of care.

Evidence-based rapid assessment and interpretation of the patient's condition

The purpose of undertaking a rapid assessment and interpretation of a patient's condition is to:

*   anticipate potential risks;
*   prevent deterioration;
*   ensure timely interventions to provide optimal outcome.

The Airway – Breathing – Circulation – Disability – Exposure 'ABCDE' approach to assessment advocated by the Resuscitation Council (UK) (2006a) provides a simple but systematic and priority-driven approach that focuses initially on assessing patient safety and then provides a focus for more in-depth assessment once the patient's safety has been established. When the ABCDE approach is combined with clinical assessment processes – including look, listen, feel, measure, monitor, collate evidence and finally respond – you will have the basis of preliminary but detailed assessment data that can be used to communicate and collaborate with the medical team in order to achieve an effective response.

In the remainder of this chapter you will be taken through the rapid assessment process by using the core skills: Look: Listen: Feel: Measure, monitor and collate evidence: and Respond.

Each element of the process is summarised in table format and provides a working guide that you can apply to scenarios in this book and in the clinical practice. In the tables below each assessment activity is prioritised and listed using 'A-B-C-D-E'; there are columns that illustrate normal and abnormal signs and tips for drawing conclusions and taking action. It is important to note that while, for the purpose of this book, these core skills have been listed in separate tables, in practice you will be using these skills concurrently and consistently in order to manage patient care.

Look at your patient

As you approach the patient, your initial observation of them begins and your priority is to look and assess for any evidence of patient distress. Nurses often say that they only have to look at a patient to know there is something wrong: what they are actually doing is using their skills of visual perception, combined with knowledge and clinical experience to interpret a picture of the patient before them (Tait, 2009; Thompson and Dowding, 2002). These are shown in Table 1.3.

Listen to your patient, relatives and clinical staff

Once you have approached the patient, the second sense to utilise is that of listening. This includes listening for signs of a patient's physiological distress such as noisy and laboured breathing and/or signs of psychological distress such as crying. Assessment skills related to listening include the active process of gathering verbal data from the patient and/or relatives, receiving handover from clinical staff and the process of linking relevant data to form clinical judgements. These are illustrated in Table 1.4.

Feel your patient's skin and pulse

The use of touch in professional caring can be described as being involved with functional nursing activities related to physical aspects of care as well as therapeutic nursing activities related to communication and psychological care. When undertaking a rapid assessment of a patient, your priority is to focus on factors affecting circulation. This includes assessing for evidence of cardiac activity and changes to the patient's circulation. Table 1.5 focuses on the rapid assessment of skin and pulse.

Assessment data	Normal signs	Abnormal signs	Drawing conclusions/taking action
1. Are they breathing? pattern: 10–20/min.	1. Quiet regular respiratory	1. Absent breathing. Laboured breathing.	1. Is the patient breathing? Respiratory/cardiac arrest? Can the patient breathe?
2. Is there an airway obstruction?	2. Rise and fall of the chest.	2. No rise and fall of the chest or abdomen, frothy sputum, choking behaviour, coughing.	2. Is the breathing laboured? Is the chest rising evenly? Is there sputum? If so, what is the volume, consistency and colour?
3. Skin colour and texture?	3. Skin is pink or brown with pink mucosa.	3. Skin pale, grey/blue tinge. Lips and mucosa pink, pale blue or purple.	3. Is their skin pale, red, flushed, cyanosed; is the skin dry and flaky?
4. Trauma/injury?	4. No signs of physical damage to the person, comfortable in any position. Calm facial expression.	4. Facial grimacing, frowning. Visible bruising, physical trauma, foreign object in the person, distortion of limbs, abnormal movement of the chest, immobility.	4. Are there signs of injury, trauma, and blood loss? Are they unable to tolerate certain positions such as sitting, standing, lying?
5. Behaviour?	5. Is conscious and able to respond.	5. Unconscious, eyes open to pain, agitated, drowsy, slack facial expression, drooling and tongue hanging out.	5. Are they agitated, anxious, AVPU score, is there evidence of facial or limb paralysis?
6. Is there evidence of contamination?	6. No evidence of toxic substances, foreign objects in the locality.	6. Visible evidence of toxic substances, insects or other contaminants.	6. Is there evidence of toxic substances? Does the patient have red wheals on their skin?

Table 1.3: Quick guide to rapid assessment and response to clinical deterioration: Look: Airway, Breathing, Circulation, Disability, Exposure

Assessment data	Normal signs	Abnormal signs	Drawing conclusions/taking action
1. Is the breathing noisy?	1. Quiet respiratory pattern.	1. Noisy breathing, respiratory strider, wheeze, rattle.	1. Noisy breathing is always abnormal! Are they wheezy (asthma), bubbling frothy sputum (pulmonary oedema), rattling noise in their chest from sputum?
2. Do they have a cough?	2. No cough.	2. Cough: dry, chesty, productive. Sputum green, yellow, orange, black, thick tenacious, copious amounts (fills a tissue in one cough).	2. Are they expectorating sputum when they cough? If so, how much and what colour is it?
3. Have you listened to the patient's or relative's story of events?	3. Patient is able to give you a clear account of their problem and history.	3. Patient is unable to respond, unconscious, confused and unable to give appropriate answers. A relative or others are able to give an account of the events.	3. Always listen and be alert to information regardless of the source: it may be important!
4. Do you know the patient?	4. The patient has a named nurse.	4. The patient is registered 'do not resuscitate'; patient has been admitted in the last 24 hours, patient is not known by the staff.	4. Do you know this patient and their situation? Are they for active treatment?
5. Have you listened to the past and recent history?	5. Patient recent and past history available.	5. A new admission, no previous history available.	5. If you know nothing about the patient or their history, then assume that the patient is for active treatment and resuscitation.

Table 1.4: Quick guide to rapid assessment and response to clinical deterioration: Listen: Airway, Breathing, Circulation

Assessment data	Normal signs	Abnormal signs	Drawing conclusions/taking action
1. Skin?	1. Skin is warm to touch and well perfused.	1. Skin is cold, hot, dry and/or flaky, damaged. Presence of deformity.	1. Is the skin cold, warm, moist, clammy, dry, dry and flaky? Can you feel any evidence of deformity?
2. Pulse?	2. Pulse is present and regular. Pulses present in the peripheral pulse points.	2. Carotid pulse is absent. Pulse is weak and thready, full and bounding, irregular. Pulse is absent or altered in one or more of the following: pedal, radial, femoral, carotid, apex.	2. Is there a pulse? Is there cardiac output? Is the pulse weak and faint, full and bounding? Can you feel the radial, pedal, carotid femoral pulses? How does this relate to the reason for the patient's admission?

Table 1.5: Quick guide to rapid assessment and response to clinical deterioration: Feel: Airway, Breathing, Circulation, Disability, Exposure

Measure and collate evidence of clinical change

The core assessment skills of 'Look: Listen: Feel' can be completed within a few minutes of meeting the patient. The process of measuring and collating evidence for clinical change involves bringing together the objective data that can be collected on a patient through the assessment of vital signs, blood glucose, fluid and electrolyte balance, and other relevant investigations. According to Adam et al. (2010) there is strong evidence to suggest that changes in respiratory rate are associated with clinical deterioration, along with a decline in patient oxygen saturation levels, changes in pulse and blood pressure, and level of consciousness. It is at this stage that evidence of your concerns becomes apparent and, if necessary, triggers the next step. See Table 1.6.

Communicating and collaborating with patients, relatives and staff to achieve appropriate and timely interventions

Risk assessment is a continuous process. If, however, you are concerned about your patient and you wish to seek advice or help, the next stage of the process is to communicate your concerns to the relevant person or team using the recognition and response bundles (NICE, 2007a) referred to in Table 1.2.

- If you have a clinical concern about the patient and the data indicates the patient to be at a low risk, then increase the frequency of the observations and monitor the patient.
- If you have a clinical concern about the patient and the data indicates the patient to be at a medium risk, then contact the patient's medical team initially and if necessary contact the critical care outreach team.
- If you have a clinical concern about the patient and the data indicates the patient to be at a high risk, then contact the critical care outreach team urgently.

See Table 1.7.

When communicating with the medical team or critical care outreach team it is vital that the date, time and nature of your concern are identified and documented. It is this process of documentation that provides a time line and audit trail for the review of practice. SBAR is a structured communication tool that has been recommended by the Institute for Health Care Improvement (IHI, 2011a) and NICE (2007a) as a framework for improving inter-professional communication and patient safety. According to Dayton and Henriksen (2007) SBAR works because it provides a shared and logical structure for communicating core details of a patient's situation either verbally or through written communication. The tool can be used for urgent and non-urgent communication and as such offers a standardised tool for communicating clinical information.

SBAR is an abbreviation for 'Situation: Background: Assessment: Recommendation', and as a tool it meets the quality requirements for safe and effective clinical documentation of care.

Assessment data	Normal signs	Abnormal signs	Drawing conclusions/taking action
1. Respiration (R)	1. R: 10–20/min	1. R: <10, >20	• Assess the patient in context: Are you concerned about your patient?
2. Pulse (P)	2. P: 60–100/min	2. P: <60, >100	• Is there evidence to support this from 'Look: Listen: Feel: Measure'?
3. Blood pressure (BP)	3. BP: 100/70–140/90	3. BP: <100/70, >140/90	• If so, what information is there and can you see a pattern or trend in deterioration?
4. Oxygen saturation (SaO$_2$)	4. SaO$_2$: 95%	4. SaO$_2$: <95%	• Has the track and trigger score changed?
5. Arterial blood gas analysis (ABG)	5. ABG: pH: 7.35–7.45; PaO$_2$: 11.5–13.5kPa; PaCO$_2$: 4.5–6.0kPa; HCO$_3$: 24–27mmol/l	5. ABG: • Respiratory acidosis: pH: <7.35; PaCO$_2$: > 6.0kPa. • Respiratory alkalosis: pH: >7.45; PaCO$_2$ <4.9kPa. • Metabolic acidosis: pH: <7.35; HCO$_3$: <22mmol/L. • Metabolic alkalosis: pH: >7.45; HCO$_3$: >26 mmol/L.	• Is there evidence of sepsis? (See Chapter 7.)
6. Pain score	6. Pain managed effectively.	6. Elevated pain score	
7. Level of consciousness (LOC)	7. APVU score: A; GCS score: 15	7. APVU score indicating < alert. GCS: <15	
8. Electrocardiogram (ECG)	8. Sinus rhythm.	8. Evidence of any abnormal-looking complexes and irregularities in rate.	

Table 1.6: Quick guide to rapid assessment and response to clinical deterioration: Measure: Airway; Breathing; Circulation; Disability; Exposure

Continued

Assessment data	Normal signs	Abnormal signs	Drawing conclusions/taking action
9. Central venous pressure (CVP)	9. Mid-axilla: 2–6mmHg/ 5–10cm H2O	9. Mid-axilla: • Hypovolaemia. CVP: <2–6mmHg; • Hypervolaemia/cardiac failure. CVP: >2–6mmHg	
10. Urine output	10. ≥0.5ml/kg body weight/hr (≥ 1000ml/24hrs)	10. Urine output: • Oliguria (acute renal failure): <0.5ml/kg body weight/hr; • Polyurea (diabetes, diabetes insipidus). Negative urine balance in spite of rigorous fluid replacement.	
11. Fluid balance	11. Fluid balance should be equal (=) based on a minimum input of 2L/24hrs	11. Fluid balance < or > = based on a minimum input of 2L/24hrs.	
12. Blood results: glucose, urea and creatinine electrolytes, microbiology	12. Blood results: glucose: 4–8mmol/L; urea: 3.5–6.5mmol/L; creatinine: 60–120 micromol/L; Na: 135–145mmol/L; K: 3.5–4.5 mmol/L; Mg: 1.25–2.5mmol/L; Cl: 95–108mmol/L; no evidence of sepsis.	12. Blood results: glucose: < or > 4–8mmol/L; urea: < or > 3.5–6.5mmol/L; creatinine: > 60–120micromol/L; Na: < or > 135–145mmol/L; K: < or > 3.5–4.5mmol/L; Mg: < or > 1.25–2.5mmol/L; Cl: < or > 95–108mmol/L; sepsis screening positive.	

Table 1.6: Continued

Activity	Assessment data	Normal signs	Abnormal signs	Drawing conclusions/ taking action
Monitor	1. Minimum 12 hourly to maximum every 15 minutes depending on the severity of the patient's illness. 2. Track and trigger score.	1. Risk assessment.	1. The monitoring of your patient should increase in frequency if you become concerned or notice any change in their condition. 2. The track and trigger score is indicating low/medium or high risk.	1. Are there changes in the physiological measures using track and trigger scoring? 2. Is your patient at risk of deterioration? 3. Have you responded?
Respond	1. Communicate with the clinical team using the SBAR tool.	1. Communicate and document ongoing patient care. 2. Continue to risk assess.	1. Recognise and respond to any concerns or clinical deterioration in your patient.	SBAR tool: 1. What is the *situation* (reason for your call)? 2. What is the clinical *background*? 3. What are the changes that have occurred in the patient *assessment* now or over time? 4. What do you suggest may be the problem? What is your *recommendation*? What do you want the clinical team to do?

Table 1.7 Quick guide to rapid assessment and response to clinical deterioration: Monitor and Respond

Situation: Identify yourself, your location and the patient. Describe the problem, your concern and reason for calling.

Background: Provide the patient's reason for admission, diagnosis and relevant history.

Assessment: Provide both your subjective concerns and objective data. Offer a provisional diagnosis of the problem or clarify your concern.

Recommendations: Explain what you need, when and where.

In the example in the table below, Molly Jones has been identified as being at risk and the essential details have been passed on to the medical registrar in charge of Molly's care. She is considered to be at moderate risk of further deterioration and needs to be monitored closely. After being seen by the registrar, Molly had blood taken for microbiological culture, was commenced

Date and time of initial call: *21/06/11 at 19.00hrs* Date and time of response: *21/06/11 at 19.10 hrs*	Patient's name: *Molly Jones: age 80 years* Nurse's name: *Debbie Smith* Name of person called: *medical registrar (Brian James)*
Situation: Reason for the call	*I am concerned about Molly Jones; she was admitted today after falling at home; she also has a rash around her waist. The rash appears angrier in the last hour and she has become drowsier and there are changes in her vital signs.*
Background	*15-year history of polymyalgia rheumatica and temporal arteritis for which she takes prednisilone. Otherwise physically well before the fall.*
Assessment	T: *38.5*; P: *95*; R: *23*; BP: *120/80*; oxygen saturations: *94%*; Blood glucose: *7mmol/l.* Track and trigger score: *has increased from 1 to 3.* Other relevant data: *Molly has been unable to pass urine since admission.* *Molly now meets the criteria for sepsis following an increase in T, P and R (see Chapter 7).* *Molly is for active resuscitation.*
Recommendations and response	What you are requesting: Ward visit: *Yes* Telephone advice: – Prescription: – Other: *I have commenced oxygen according to her prescription and increased her observations to hourly.* Action taken and Registrar's response: *Thank you. Can you continue with the oxygen therapy and I will come and reassess the patient? Please have ready the equipment for taking blood cultures and setting up an intravenous infusion. I will be on the ward in 15 minutes. We will also need to consider if Molly needs urinary catheterisation.* Signatures: *Signed by both the staff nurse and the registrar following Molly's assessment.*

Table 1.8: Communicating concern using the SBAR approach

on an intravenous infusion and intravenous antibiotics. She had a urinary catheter inserted, and that confirmed the presence of a urine output of less than 50ml per hour; a catheter specimen of urine revealed a urinary tract infection. Molly was also diagnosed with shingles. Following 48 hours of antibiotic therapy and fluid resuscitation, Molly began to improve and was no longer considered to be at risk. She was eventually discharged home five days later.

Providing standardised and optimal care during all stages of the patient's journey

A registered nurse has a professional responsibility to ensure safe and clinically effective care in order to support an agreed patient outcome and to accurately document any changes in the patient's condition or variance from the care pathway. The adoption of a care pathways and a care bundle approach by the National Institute for Health and Clinical Excellence (NICE, 2011) has given all health care providers an opportunity to standardise practice while continuing to provide patient-focused care. The emphasis is now on you as a nurse to recognise and adopt the most clinically appropriate pathway of care, but at the same time to recognise, record and respond to any variances in the care package. In this context those variances have to be justified and evidence based. The seven points below are a useful guide to what should be provided to ensure the quality of nursing documentation (Jeffries et al., 2010).

1. Patient centred and includes extracts from the patient's description of their illness experience.
2. Reflects the objective clinical judgement of the nurse so that every statement has an objective descriptor. For example:
    a) Subjective comment: The patient seemed a bit tipsy.
    b) Objective comment: The patient was walking with an unsteady gait, his speech was slurred and his breath smelt of alcohol.
3. Contains the actual work of nurses including bio-psychosocial interventions.
4. Presented in a logical sequence.
5. Written as events occur so that it remains up to date.
6. Records all variances in care, in a clear and concise way without repetition.
7. Fulfils legal and professional requirements according to the NMC *Standards of conduct, performance and ethics* (2008).

In a busy and acute clinical setting nurses and health care professionals can easily be distracted. The safety of patients, however, should be paramount and the prevention of patient deterioration a multidisciplinary goal that can only be achieved through assessment, communication and collaboration between the patient and all professional groups.

Managing and organising care using the appropriate skill mix

The ability to know and understand your patients is dependent on you and your team having a balanced skill mix, evidence of continuity of care, effective communication channels and effective team work so that you are able to assess and respond to the patient's immediate needs in an emergency (Scott, 2003; Duffield et al., 2010).

There is a wide range of skill mix in acute care across hospitals and even in the same hospital (Scott, 2003; Duffield et al., 2010) because of changes in nurse education strategies and the loss of nursing apprentices. In acute care the number of health care assistants has increased at a faster rate than that of registered nurses, leading to a dilution of professionally registered nurses in the skill mix (Scott, 2003). Furthermore, staffing levels often vary because of staff sickness, unexpected patient turnover and the use of bank or agency nurses.

Within this climate of change in models of health care provision, there is evidence to support the use of a collaborative team approach to care (Royal College of Nursing, 2003; Zwarenstein et al., 2009). A team may consist of all the providers of care for a group of patients, including nurses, health care assistants, medical staff and other health professionals. Nonetheless, the focus should remain on patient-centred care where continuity of care is provided by the team, with each team member ensuring effective communication. Task-based team nursing, where management of care is based on a series of tasks rather than focusing on patient need, should be avoided, as this has been found to reduce the quality of care (Fairbrother et al., 2010).

In the activity below you have a chance to practise rapid assessment and management of a patient.

Activity 1.2   *Decision-making*

Gladys, aged 63 years, is normally a healthy and active grandmother. She takes a beta blocker to manage hypertension. Gladys has a two-day history of vomiting and muscle weakness, following which she developed pain on passing urine. Her GP diagnosed a urinary tract infection secondary to a viral infection and prescribed amoxicillin. Two days later Gladys was admitted to the medical admission unit with a history of falls and confusion, and you are asked to admit and assess her.

1. What knowledge and skills would you use to assess Gladys on admission?
2. On assessment the following data were collected regarding her condition:
   a) **Tachypnoea** with a rate of 28/min, SaO_2 86%.
   b) Skin is pale and dry.
   c) Confused with a GCS of 6/15.
   d) T 37.8°C.
   e) Pulse 98 BPM.
   f) BP 110/40 mmHg.
   g) Has not passed urine for 12 hours.
3. What concerns would you have?
4. What will you do about your concerns?

There are sample answers to this question at the end of the chapter.

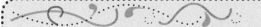

Chapter summary

Within this chapter we have introduced you to the skills and processes involved in the rapid assessment of and response to deteriorating patients. The core skills focus on risk assessment, prevention and timely intervention of care, and the tables included have been designed to provide you with an aide memoire that you can apply to the patient examples in the remainder of the book.

Activities: brief outline answers

Activity 1.2: Risk assessment and clinical decision making (page 22)

The knowledge and skills you would use relate to clinical assessment and in particular rapid assessment skills. These include using 'ABCDE' as a guide: look at the patient; listen to the patient, family, handover from other staff, listen for physiological signs of distress; feel the patient's skin and note any abnormal signs; measure the patient's physiological signs. Interpret the clinical signs and assess the findings against the normal range. Assess the degree of concern guided by the local track and trigger score on the assessment sheet.

Your concerns for this lady should focus on the following.

- Increased respiratory rate with a lower than normal SaO_2 suggests respiratory distress and requires immediate action: call for help from a senior member of staff and administer oxygen guided by the local protocol.
- Confusion due to a number of possible factors, including hypoxaemia, dehydration, electrolyte imbalance (see Chapter 8).
- Pyrexia.
- Haemodynamic insufficiency – low BP and fast pulse (see Chapter 6).
- This lady is very sick. Her trigger score would be in the high risk range and she needs immediate assessment from the critical care outreach team.

Gladys was assessed and transferred for treatment in ICU. You can pick up her story in Chapter 3.

Further reading

Royal College of Nursing (RCN) (2004) *Nursing assessment of older people: RCN Tool Kit.* London: RCN.

This resource provides general guidance and tools for assessing older people and offers useful background detail on collaborative assessment processes.

Rushforth, H. (2009) *Nursing assessment made incredibly easy.* London: Wolters Kluwer/Lippincott Williams and Wilkins.

This book provides information on detailed systematic assessment of all clinical situations and is a useful revision guide to assessment skills.

Useful websites

www.resus.org.uk/pages/dnar.htm

This resource provides information and guidance by the Resuscitation Council on ethical decisions related to resuscitation.

Chapter 2
The breathless patient

Jane James with Julie Wickland

NMC Standards for Pre-registration Nursing Education

This chapter will address the following competencies:

Domain 3: Nursing practice and decision-making

Generic competencies:
7. All nurses must be able to recognise and interpret signs of normal and deteriorating mental and physical health and respond promptly to maintain or improve the health and comfort of the service user, acting to keep them and others safe.

Field-specific competencies:
7.1. Adult nurses must recognise the early signs of illness in people of all ages. They must make accurate assessments and start appropriate and timely management of those who are acutely ill, at risk of clinical deterioration, or require emergency care.

NMC Essential Skills Clusters

This chapter will address the following ESCs:

Cluster: Care, compassion and communication
1. As partners in the care process, people can trust a newly registered graduate nurse to provide collaborative care based on the highest standards, knowledge and competence.

By entry to the register:
viii. Demonstrates clinical confidence through sound knowledge, skills and understanding relevant to field.
ix. Is self-aware and self-confident, knows own limitations and is able to take appropriate action.

Cluster: Organisational aspects of care
9. People can trust the newly registered graduate nurse to treat them as partners and work with them to make a holistic and systematic assessment of their needs; to develop a personalised plan that is based on mutual understanding and respect for their individual situation promoting health and well-being, minimising risk of harm and promoting their safety at all times.

By entry to the register:
xx. Acts autonomously and appropriately when faced with sudden deterioration in people's physical or psychological condition or emergency situations, abnormal vital signs, collapse, cardiac arrest, self-harm, extremely challenging behaviour, attempted suicide.
xxi. Measures documents and interprets vital signs and acts autonomously and appropriately on findings.

Chapter aims

By the end of this chapter, you should be able to:

*   identify causes of breathlessness;
*   describe the clinical features of breathlessness in relation to type I and II respiratory failure, pneumonia, chronic obstructive pulmonary disease (COPD) and asthma, and the clinical implications for the patient;
*   demonstrate awareness of how to undertake respiratory assessment;
*   diagnose and differentiate between possible causes of patient deterioration and identify most appropriate interventions;
*   reflect on clinical examples illustrated in the chapter and relate to your own clinical practice.

Introduction

Case study: Cardiac failure

Susan had been allocated a small caseload of patients to visit while on her final community placement. One of her patients was 76-year-old Charlie Morris, who had been having a chronic leg wound redressed twice weekly. When Susan arrived at his house on her second visit, she found Mr Morris sitting in a chair dressed in his pyjamas. He said he was having trouble getting going and was very tired because he had not slept very well. His wife added that he had woken several times during the night short of breath, had sat on the edge of the bed and asked her to open the window. He seemed better once morning came. Mr Morris said that this happened to him sometimes, but not usually this bad. He normally rested and felt better after a while.

When Susan went to look at Mr Morris's wound, she found the leg of his pyjamas was very tight. In helping her to access his wound, he struggled to remove his pyjamas, becoming breathless and needing time afterwards to get his breath back. Susan also found the wound bandage was constricting Mr Morris's leg, which appeared swollen; his toes were cold and pale. She wondered if she had applied the bandage too tightly on her previous visit and contacted her mentor, Bridget, to ask for advice.

Bridget called by and assessed Mr Morris. First, she checked his respirations, pulse and blood pressure, then asked questions about his regular medication and his fluid intake and output, felt both Mr Morris's ankles and listened carefully to what Mrs Morris told her. Susan was confused as to why Bridget did not seem concerned about Mr Morris's leg wound, but instead requested the GP to visit, saying that she thought he might have an exacerbation of his heart failure.

Susan's experience highlights the fact that patients with chronic conditions often have more than one problem. Susan thought that she was visiting Mr Morris for a straightforward dressing change, but his other health problems were more serious at that time.

The fact that Mr Morris was feeling tired and lethargic was not simply due to a poor night's sleep. The reason why his sleep was disturbed was significant in that he was waking up from sleep feeling short of breath, and this happened several times. The fact that the degree of breathlessness related to physical exertion and speaking was also worthy of note.

When Bridget heard Mrs Morris's story and saw that to a degree Mr Morris was still breathless at rest and had swollen legs, she recognised some important indicators and knew from her experience that it could be a worsening of Mr Morris's heart failure. Susan had only seen Mr Morris once previously and had been concentrating on being professional and doing the dressing correctly. She was glad that she had contacted her mentor, even though her reason was misdirected.

Susan visited Mr Morris to do a dressing but found that he was tired and breathless. His main problem was not his wound but related to his heart. What can we learn from this?

The important messages in Susan's story are these.

- Take every opportunity in all clinical settings to assess your patients holistically and systematically (see Chapter 1); assimilate your findings and keep an open mind.
- Listen carefully to your patient's complaints or concerns about things such as breathlessness that affect their daily activities, as these are often significant.
- If you are concerned about your patient, seek advice and support according to local risk assessment protocol (see Chapter 1).
- The seat of the problem may not necessarily be what you think, and breathlessness alone or combined with other symptoms needs further exploration.

This chapter gives an overview of the possible causes of breathlessness and examines in detail the care of patients suffering with breathlessness related to: 1) heart failure; 2) pneumonia; 3) COPD; 4) asthma. Underlying physiology, social psychology and ethical implications of all four types of patients will be discussed in the context of risk assessment and collaborative management and care.

The chapter begins with an explanation of breathlessness, leading to an overview of the knowledge and skills required to recognise, assess, prioritise and manage care for patients with breathlessness. This chapter introduces the need for respiratory support and the concept of arterial blood gas analysis, but these are discussed in detail in Chapters 3 and 10.

Breathlessness

Breathing is vital for life and is part of the mechanism depended upon to supply oxygen to the tissues. All cells in the human body require a continuous supply of oxygen or they die. As oxygen is used, carbon dioxide is produced as a waste product. While it is important for the body to take in oxygen, it is also important to remove the carbon dioxide at the same rate that oxygen is supplied. Essentially, this is respiration, and it contributes to maintaining homeostasis – a state of balance and stability within the cells to keep them working. If the cells receive insufficient amounts of oxygen, they become hypoxic. This state is known as tissue hypoxia and can cause increased acid production, resulting in cell death (Kumar and Clark, 2001). Likewise, if the carbon dioxide is not removed efficiently, it builds up in the blood (CO_2 retention) creating hypercarbia and has the effect of increasing blood acid levels.

Acidity and alkalinity, body temperature and fluid levels are also involved in homeostasis. All of these factors can be controlled to achieve the narrow range of normality required, by adaptations in response from various body systems (Porth, 1998). The respiratory system is involved in controlling and responding to all the aforementioned factors, and while respiration itself comprises four processes (Table 2.1), in the first instance, we notice our patients' bodies attempting to achieve homeostasis by changes in their breathing.

When different factors of homeostasis are disturbed and the body tries to adjust to put things back to normal (compensation), it does this initially by altering the rate and pattern of breathing.

Process	Dependent upon	Measured by	Clinical examples
Pulmonary ventilation: the movement of air in and out of the lungs.	Chemoreceptors in aorta, carotid body and medulla oblongata. Respiratory centres in the brain. Nerves: phrenic, intercostal. Muscles: diaphragm, intercostal muscles, accessory muscles. Pressure changes within thoracic cavity. Patent airways. Elasticity of lungs. Lung capacity.	Respiratory observations: rate; depth; sound; effort; volumes.	1. Jean has Guillain Barré syndrome affecting the nerves supplying her intercostal muscles and reducing the size of her breaths. 2. John has asthma and bronchospasm, which restricts the flow of air through his airways. 3. Peter sustained broken ribs when a tree fell on him, causing pneumothorax and precluding him from taking deep breaths. 4. Diane suffered a head injury affecting her brain stem. 5. Phil was trapped in a fire and breathed in hot smoke causing pharyngeal oedema.
External respiration: the exchange of oxygen and carbon dioxide between the alveoli in the lungs and the pulmonary capillaries.	Tidal volume > physiological dead space. Fresh supply of oxygen to alveoli. Gas pressure changes (oxygen and carbon dioxide). Diffusion. Presence of blood supply (pulmonary capillaries). Proximity of pulmonary blood flow to alveoli.	Inspired/expired gas analysis.	1. Mary took an overdose of her sleeping tablets and has very shallow breaths. 2. Chris is climbing Mount Everest and developed pulmonary oedema due to lower air pressure at altitude. 3. Brian has COPD with emphysema and atelectasis. 4. Ross was recovering from hip surgery when he suffered a pulmonary embolism. 5. Sally has pneumonia and secretions have consolidated the bases of both lungs.

Table 2.1 Processes of respiration

Continued

Process	Dependent upon	Measured by	Clinical examples
Transport of gases: the carriage of oxygen from the lungs to the tissues and carbon dioxide from the tissues to the lungs in the blood.	Circulation of blood. Patency of vessels. Uninterrupted flow.	Oxygen saturations. Arterial blood gas analysis (ABG).	1. Charlie has heart failure and reduced cardiac output. 2. Trudy is anaemic after months of heavy periods. 3. Margaret had a thrombosis that lodged in her popliteal artery causing her foot to become ischaemic.
Internal respiration: the delivery of oxygen to the body cells and the collection of carbon dioxide from the cells	Gas pressure changes. Blood supply to cells. Correct environment within the cell.	ABGs – level of metabolic acidosis. Lactate levels.	1. Bob's gas fire was faulty and he suffered carbon monoxide poisoning. 2. Andy fell into the river and suffered hypothermia.

Table 2.1: Continued

So anyone who is breathless (dyspnoeic) is in the process of trying to normalise their body's internal environment. Their degree of breathlessness often indicates the severity of imbalance within their cells, and could be caused by problems with any one of the four processes involved in respiration as shown in the clinical examples in Table 2.1. These processes can be affected by other body systems as demonstrated by Mr Morris's heart failure in the case study above. As his heart failed to pump effectively, there was inadequate circulation to maintain his blood pressure and internal respiration, resulting in poor tissue oxygenation. Mr Morris's frequent episodes of breathlessness during the night resulted from his body trying to compensate.

Mr Morris also had swelling (**oedema**) of his lower legs, and this was a key indicator to Bridget that Mr Morris was retaining fluid. She knew that Mr Morris's heart was probably working harder and that his lungs might well be congested due to the increased fluid in his body, thus affecting his external respiration. When she found that he was hypotensive as well as dyspnoeic and tachycardic, she was satisfied with her assessment.

Because breathlessness can result from the body's compensation in relation to the respiratory, circulatory, neuromuscular, renal and metabolic systems, you will find breathless patients of all ages and in all clinical settings. Breathing rates change quickly in response to demands from body systems, so breathlessness is an early indicator of acute illness and should not be ignored (NICE 2007a, NPSA 2007a). In order to prevent further deterioration you need to be alert to breathless patients and undertake an initial rapid assessment using the ABCDE approach (Resuscitation Council (UK), 2006b), as outlined in Chapter 1, followed by a more detailed assessment of breathing. This needs to be combined with the clinical assessment process of 'Look: Listen: Feel: Measure', which will enable you to respond appropriately to your patients' needs in a timely manner (Smith et al., 2009).

Breathing assessment

As part of the ABCDE approach to organising rapid assessment, it is important to ensure that your patient's airway is patent before going on to assess breathing. On assessing your patients, you will be aware of several aspects of breathing, and noting these can be very useful in identifying risks and changes in your patients' conditions.

Activity 2.1   *Critical thinking*

Consider the patients in Table 2.1 and note down how many different aspects of breathing you can think of. Remember to use the 'Look: Listen: Feel: Measure' approach discussed in Chapter 1.

A table of what you could identify is given at the end of the chapter.

Bridget rapidly assessed Mr Morris when she arrived to see him. She could see that he was alert, as he replied to her when she greeted him. This also verified that his airway was clear. She could see that he was breathing and that it seemed to be fast, so she made a mental note to return to breathing assessment in more detail. Bridget confirmed signs of circulation by noting the colour and temperature of Mr Morris's skin and by quickly checking his pulse as she took his hand. Checking his blood pressure would give more detailed information later. Bridget noted

Mr Morris's answers to her brief questions, quickly assessing his level of consciousness in relation to disability, and in relation to exposure as she looked at all other areas of his body. She could see that his lower legs were swollen, but his main problem was breathlessness.

Using the 'Look: Listen: Feel: Measure' approach, Bridget went on to assess Mr Morris's breathing in more detail. She could see that he was pale and his chest was rising equally on both sides. He was breathing fast and deep. He did not look distressed, but he was using his accessory muscles (pulling his shoulders up and pushing his abdomen out). Breathing looked hard work for him and his nostrils were flaring slightly on inspiration. This informed Bridget that he was trying to get more air into his lungs and that he might be short of oxygen.

Bridget went on to listen, and she could hear the air moving in and out of Mr Morris's nose. It was audible as she knelt next to him, but was not noisy. She then listened with a stethoscope to the front and back of his chest. She moved her stethoscope systematically over the chest, listening at specific points identified in Figure 2.1.

On listening with the stethoscope, Bridget could hear the air moving in and out of Mr Morris's lungs as he breathed normally. She also asked him to take some deeper breaths in order to improve the quality of the breath sounds she could hear. There were crackles all over his chest at the end of inspiration and a faint wheeze on expiration. This suggested to her that he had fluid accumulating in the tissues of his lungs (pulmonary oedema), which would obstruct external respiration.

When Bridget put her hands flat on Mr Morris's chest, she felt his chest expanding equally on the left and the right and she could feel the movement of fluid as Mr Morris breathed in and out. His skin felt cool and clammy, suggesting that his peripheral circulation was poor.

Bridget counted Mr Morris's breaths (in and out) for one minute to measure his respiratory rate at 32 breaths per minute (bpm). She also noted that he could speak four or five words between breaths. She had been very mindful to ask open questions in order to measure this, but subsequently asked only closed questions to avoid additional undue breathlessness. Her hand-held oxygen saturation monitor told her that his oxygen saturations (SaO_2) were 94%, indicating that he was just achieving the target range of 94–98% recommended by O'Driscoll et al. (2008).

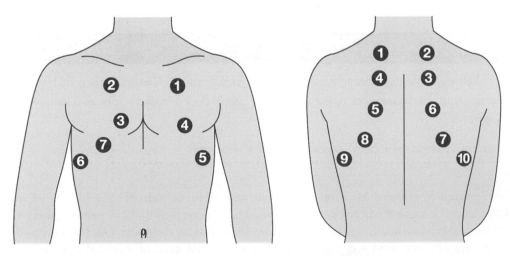

Figure 2.1: Position and sequence for stethoscope placement when listening to breathing sounds as shown by numbered dots

Activity 2.2	*Evidence-based practice and research*

Visit the 3M™ Littman® Stethoscopes website education page below and follow the link 'About Stethoscopes' to find information about the components of a stethoscope and how to use it.

> http://solutions.3m.com/wps/portal/3M/en_US/3M-Littmann/stethoscope/
> littmann-learning-institute/

After gaining consent, practise the 'Look: Listen: Feel: Measure' approach to performing a respiratory assessment on a well person and on your patients with breathlessness.

Practise using your stethoscope to listen to the areas of the chest identified on Figure 2.1. Make notes and compare your findings.

There is a link on the website to 'Heart & Lung Sounds'. Follow this link to hear some different breathing sounds to compare with your findings.

As this answer is based on your own observations, there is no outline answer at the end of the chapter.

Following assessment of Mr Morris's breathing, Bridget completed her assessment of his circulation by feeling and measuring his pulse rate and blood pressure. She looked over the rest of his body (exposure), feeling where necessary. Bridget also considered other information she had gained on questioning Mr and Mrs Morris and her previous knowledge of his medical history. She recognised that tachycardia, hypotension and leg oedema supported her respiratory assessment to conclude that Mr Morris had worsening heart failure. She now needed to get him the required treatment and care.

Why is oxygen important?

Scenario: Pneumonia

Imagine you are working in the Accident and Emergency Department (A&E) when Sally French, a 38-year-old physical education teacher is brought in with breathing difficulties, pain in her chest and confusion.

The paramedics report that she has had influenza-like symptoms for the past four days and seems to be getting worse. They give details of their assessment and interventions: due to her tachypnoea, respiratory distress and oxygen saturations of 90%, they have given high flow oxygen via a non-rebreathing mask (Figure 2.2), and inserted an intravenous cannula into her left hand.

You see that Mrs French is sitting up and talking, but she appears weak and unable to support herself. You have difficulty getting her to concentrate on what you are telling her and asking her to do. Your mentor asks you to do her observations while she goes to get the doctor, and you find that Mrs French has a temperature of 38.6°C, her pulse rate is 122 bpm, respiratory rate is

Figure 2.2: A non-rebreathing mask with reservoir bag. The reservoir fills with oxygen and the mask delivers up to 70% oxygen. These masks are used for patients who are in severe respiratory distress.

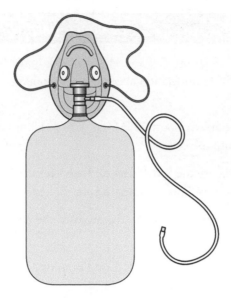

38 bpm. She is still wearing the non-rebreathing oxygen mask that the paramedics gave her, and this is delivering oxygen to her at around 70%. Mrs French's oxygen saturations are now 92% and her blood pressure is 105/48 mmHg (normal adult blood pressure 100–140mmHg systolic, 60–90mmHg diastolic).

Activity 2.3   *Decision-making*

Look carefully at Table 1.1 (on pp7–8), and identify which level of critical care Sally French falls into and give your reasons for your decision. Then, using Table 1.2 (p10), apply the admission, recognition and response bundles of care to Sally.

An outline of how these apply to Sally is given at the end of the chapter.

Your main concern for Sally is that her SaO_2 levels are too low and have improved only marginally from 90% to 92% since receiving high-flow oxygen at about 70% via the non-rebreathing mask. These levels are worrying because the target saturations for an adult are 94–98%, and in health these are normally achieved without added oxygen (O'Driscoll et al., 2008). It is worth considering the accuracy of the reading, but you note that she is still dyspnoeic, tachypnoeic, tachycardic and confused. These are signs of low blood oxygen levels (hypoxaemia). From your rapid assessment and the track and trigger score, you can calculate that she is at high risk of deterioration.

Sally is already receiving high-flow oxygen and you must consider other ways of improving her oxygenation because she has not responded sufficiently, she needs more oxygen delivered to her body cells and you cannot increase the oxygen further by face mask. Despite her blood pressure being borderline low, it is important for her to sit as upright as possible in order to maximise her pulmonary ventilation (Table 2.1). Gravity helps to increase lung compliance (elasticity) and lung volume by allowing her accessory muscles to work more easily, thus enabling larger breaths for less effort (Fleming and Todd, 1998). Breath size is important as not all inspired air reaches the alveoli. No gas exchange takes place in the nasal passages, trachea, bronchi and bronchioles, known as anatomical dead space, and these constitute approximately 150ml of inhaled air. It is more effective for Sally to increase her breath size, known as tidal volume (the volume of air inhaled and exhaled at each breath), than her respiratory rate (the number of breaths taken within a set amount of time, typically 60 seconds); she is already breathing very fast and is getting tired. She needs to get more oxygen into her blood to cope with the demands of her body cells. The medical team need to perform further investigations to give an indication of how this might be achieved. These should include a chest X-ray to give a picture of lung inflation and blood tests for full blood count (FBC), urea and electrolytes (U&E), liver function tests (LFT), arterial blood gas analysis (ABG) and blood cultures. Together these will give indications of blood oxygen carrying capacity (haemoglobin from FBC), renal function (U&E levels), hydration (U&E levels plus haematocrit from FBC), presence of and response to infection (blood cultures and white cell count from FBC) and Sally's ability to exchange inspired oxygen for carbon dioxide (ABG). Arterial blood gas analysis will also indicate the acidity of Sally's arterial blood.

Scenario

Things happen very quickly from this point. Your mentor returns with the doctor and blood is taken to be tested for FBC, U&E, LFT, ABG and blood cultures to rule out causes such as poisoning or renal failure, and to confirm suspected infection as a cause of Sally's respiratory distress and altered consciousness. Intravenous fluids are commenced and a portable chest X-ray performed as well as a 12-lead electrocardiograph. The anaesthetist who is on call reviews Mrs French and decides that she should be quickly transferred to the High Dependency Unit with a diagnosis of type I respiratory failure secondary to community-acquired pneumonia. She needs respiratory support to improve her oxygenation, and close monitoring of her ABGs, breathing and consciousness. Temperature, heart rate and rhythm, blood pressure, oxygen saturations and fluid balance will also be monitored and recorded, as well as any pain.

How did Sally become so ill so quickly when she is so young and usually very fit? Sally has been suffering with influenza-like symptoms, most probably from a virulent infection of her upper airways. Bacteria have been aspirated into her lungs during breathing, where they have caused inflammation of the bronchioles and alveoli. The air spaces have filled with exudate (escaping fluid containing cell debris and pus), which in turn filled with white blood cells and fibrin to create a solid mass. This is consolidation (Wheeldon, 2009), which blocks inhaled oxygen from contact with the alveolar surface, thus restricting external respiration.

Sally has localised, sharp chest pain known as pleuritic pain, which results from inflammation spreading to the pleura, restricting her ability to take deep breaths. Combined with the inefficient external respiration, she has quickly become hypoxaemic and breathless. Despite her young age and usual health, Sally's defence mechanisms are failing to cope with the virulence of the infection. Without intervention to control the infection, clear secretions and correct her poor oxygenation, Sally is at serious risk of death from pneumonia and respiratory failure. Lim et al. (2009) recommend the CURB65 score to ascertain risk from community-acquired pneumonia. One point is awarded for each symptom.

- C – confusion of new onset.
- U – urea level > 7mmol/litre.
- R – respiratory rate > 30 breaths per minute.
- B – blood pressure: systolic < 90mmHg or diastolic < 60mmHg.
- 65 years of age or more.

A score of 3 or more indicates high risk of death and the need for treatment in hospital with a minimum of 12-hourly medical review, while a score of 4 or 5 requires the patient to receive intensive care (Lim et al., 2009).

From the nursing assessment we can see that Sally scores a minimum of 3, and following blood results indicating her urea level, she may score 4, confirming the need for level 2 care.

The clinical examination and chest X-ray confirm Sally's diagnosis of pneumonia, and the blood test results indicate how her body is responding and coping with the infection. The ABG analysis gives important information about her blood acidity or alkalinity (pH), levels of oxygen (PaO_2), carbon dioxide ($PaCO_2$) and bicarbonate levels (involved in CO_2 carriage), which are detailed in Table 2.2. The information is relevant to diagnosing the extent of her respiratory failure and shows the degree of deviation from normal. It also gives an accurate arterial oxygen saturation reading. This indicates her respiratory status and metabolic environment (how her cells are working) and gauges the body's ability to maintain homeostasis. Factors other than respiration and gas exchange contribute to this and will be discussed in more detail in Chapter 7.

pH	7.37	(7.35–7.45)
$PaCO_2$	5.2	(4.5–6.0kPa)
PaO_2	7.8	(10.0–13.3kPa)
HCO_3	21	(22–26mmol/L)
Base excess	−1.4	(−2–+2)
SaO_2	91%	(>95%)

Table 2.2: Sally's ABG result with normal values shown in brackets

Types of respiratory failure

Type I respiratory failure is characterised by:

- PaO_2 less than 8 kilopascals (kPa);
- low or normal $PaCO_2$.

It is also known as hypoxaemic respiratory failure and can progress to type II respiratory failure if not treated.

Type II respiratory failure is characterised by:

- PaO_2 less than 8 kPa;
- $PaCO_2$ more than 5.5 kPa (hypercarbia);
- respiratory acidosis.

Type II respiratory failure is also known as ventilatory respiratory failure.

Type I respiratory failure

Case study

Sally's ABG results show that the pH is normal, but tending towards low, her PaCO$_2$ is normal and her PaO$_2$ is low, confirming type I respiratory failure.

Her bicarbonate level is also a little low.

Sally has type I respiratory failure indicated by hypoxaemia. This must be treated to prevent progression to type II respiratory failure and the risk of tissue hypoxia, whereby insufficient oxygen is available for cell metabolism. Without adequate levels of oxygen for aerobic cell metabolism, anaerobic metabolism begins, thus producing lactic acid. Anaerobic metabolism is less efficient, and if prolonged, cells begin to swell and cell death can occur (Kumar and Clark, 2001).

Sally is already trying to compensate by breathing faster and trying to increase her pulmonary ventilation. She is receiving as much oxygen as can be given to her via oxygen mask and her SaO$_2$ readings of 92% and her confusion tell us that her body is failing to compensate. She needs intravenous antibiotics to treat the infection, and additional interventions such as humidification and nebulisers to loosen the viscous secretions that are blocking external respiration (O'Driscoll et al., 2008). If her cough is too weak to expectorate the thick sputum, Sally may need chest physiotherapy. If her condition does not improve and she becomes more tired, she may need respiratory support by non-invasive ventilation (NIV) or invasive positive pressure ventilation (IPPV) in the intensive care unit (see Chapter 3). For this reason, it is important to continually monitor Sally using the 'Look: Listen: Feel: Measure' approach. Her temperature, pulse, respiratory rate, blood pressure, mental state and SaO$_2$ against inspired oxygen should be closely observed and recorded (Lim et al., 2009). Any changes should be reported immediately to prompt a timely response.

You must ensure that measurements recorded are accurate to facilitate administration of the most appropriate treatment and care for Sally. Accurate monitoring of SaO$_2$ requires good peripheral perfusion, which can be assessed by measuring capillary refill. This is the time taken in seconds for colour to return after compressing a finger nail bed (you could practise this on your own finger nail). Capillary refill should be used as part of holistic assessment, although its value is sometimes questioned. In altered pathophysiology states such as peripheral vascular disease, results can mislead interpretation (Creed and Spiers, 2010). Oxygen saturations reliability can be affected by poor peripheral perfusion, anaemia, hypothermia, false or painted nails, bright environmental lights or incorrect probe positioning (Creed et al., 2010).

Because Sally is acutely ill, her peripheral perfusion may be compromised, affecting the accuracy of her SaO$_2$ reading. The reading is most significant when considered against the inspired oxygen percentage. A low reading recorded on breathing room air is less worrying than a low reading on high-flow oxygen. As Sally is receiving high-flow oxygen, it is important to check her ABGs again to evaluate the effectiveness of any treatment and care. Results should be considered alongside other findings from clinical assessment.

Activity 2.4   *Evidence-based practice and research*

In clinical practice where an oxygen saturations monitor with finger probe is available, ask your mentor if you and a fellow student can experiment to test the accuracy of oxygen saturations measurement on a healthy person (each other). You may also be able to do this in your university clinical skills laboratory if you ask your teacher. Apply the following variances.

- Apply a blood pressure cuff.
- Hold the arm up in the air for a few minutes.
- Apply nail polish.
- Shine a bright light close to the probe.

Note the variations in results of these actions and consider how these things apply to your patients.

As this answer is based on your own observations, there is no outline answer at the end of the chapter.

Type II respiratory failure

Case study: Chronic obstructive pulmonary disease

Paul, a student nurse, was asked to look after 64-year-old Brian Carter who was known to have COPD and previous type II respiratory failure. He was well known on the ward, having been an inpatient on several previous occasions. Three days ago he was admitted with an infected exacerbation of COPD. Following medical review, Brian was prescribed care including intravenous antibiotics, nebulisers, steroid therapy and oxygen at 24% via a venturi device (Figure 2.3) to keep his oxygen saturations above 92%.

Paul went to do Brian's observations and found that he looked quite uncomfortable. On further ABCDE assessment he found Brian's respiratory rate was 36 bpm and his oxygen saturations were reading 88% on his ear probe. His pulse rate was 127 bpm and his blood pressure was 98/52 mmHg. Paul noticed that Brian's fingers were slightly blue and his nose and lips were also rather dusky coloured. Paul tried to comfort Brian and asked how he was feeling, but his answers were difficult to hear because he seemed so short of breath and sounded wheezy. Brian looked as if he was working hard to breathe, pulling his chest up by his shoulders and breathing through pursed lips while his oxygen mask hung around his neck. He looked frightened and his hand was shaking as he reached out for a glass of water.

From Paul's assessment based upon 'Look: Listen: Feel: Measure', we can deduce that Brian is in respiratory distress. This is a serious situation with risk of further deterioration if appropriate action is not taken. Brian is struggling to get air into his lungs, and his oxygen saturation levels are too low, suggesting hypoxaemia and respiratory failure, but without ABG analysis to indicate Brian's $PaCO_2$ levels we do not know whether Brian is in type I or type II respiratory failure. Brian is, however, showing signs that he is in type II respiratory failure. Paul noticed the tachycardia under circulation assessment and under exposure should find dilation of Brian's

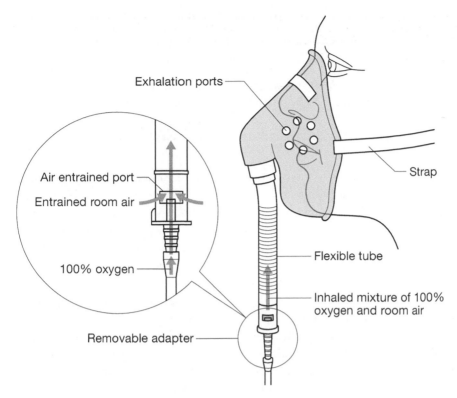

Figure 2.3: Venturi device used to administer controlled oxygen

peripheral veins and hand tremor, which are due to the effects of hypercarbia on the central vascular system and central nervous system (Green et al., 2003). Paul now needs to organise his findings to enable him to prioritise the actions he will take in order to reduce the risk of Brian deteriorating further.

As a student nurse it is important that he gets help to deal with this situation, but Paul should not leave Brian alone. He can summon his mentor by use of the bedside emergency call bell. The aim is to make breathing easier for Brian, thus improving his oxygenation and reducing his carbon dioxide levels. Considering the different phases of respiration, Paul is able to help with pulmonary ventilation and the supply of oxygen, but is unable to control other respiratory processes.

Case study

Paul explained to Brian what he was going to do and summoned his mentor. He sat Brian more upright by using the profiling action of the bed. He helped Brian to take some sips of water and made sure that the oxygen was flowing through the mask correctly, then replaced it over Brian's nose and mouth. He checked the accuracy of the oxygen saturations probe by repositioning it and continued to observe Brian's breathing effort, rate and depth. When his mentor arrived, Paul asked if he should increase the oxygen in view of Brian's breathlessness and low oxygen saturation readings, but he was advised not to. Instead he was asked to give 2 litres of oxygen via nasal cannulae while giving Brian an air-driven nebuliser. The mentor asked Paul to stay with Brian to

> reassure him and to make sure that he breathed in all the nebulised liquid. Paul's mentor also adjusted the bed so that it formed a chair shape. She asked Paul to call her when the nebuliser started to splutter.
>
> After some time and two further nebulisers, Brian's breathing slowed down and he looked more comfortable. The physiotherapist helped him to have a good cough. He expectorated large amounts of thick green–yellow sputum.

Why did Paul's mentor insist on these interventions for Brian? Sitting Brian upright would immediately make a difference to his pulmonary ventilation (see Table 2.1) by enabling larger breaths for less effort. Lowering his legs and making the bed into a chair shape reduces intra-abdominal pressure, thus allowing more space for chest expansion. As with Sally, it is more effective for Brian to increase his breath size than his respiratory rate, thus promoting better intake of oxygen and allowing exhalation of carbon dioxide. Brian may have felt anxious and acutely aware of the effort required to breathe, so it was important that Paul stayed to help and reassure him. The simple act of helping Brian take sips of water relieved the stress of discomfort from a dry mouth, caused by mouth breathing and the use of oxygen.

Once Paul had improved Brian's pulmonary ventilation, quickly checking and replacing Brian's oxygen mask over his nose and mouth would ensure that Brian was receiving the prescribed level of oxygen. Paul could not know how long Brian had been without the extra oxygen, and so it was sensible to check and reposition the oxygen saturations probe to ensure a good pulse was sensed, thus assuring accuracy of the reading. Paul could then also check that the displayed pulse rate corresponded to Brian's palpated pulse rate.

Even though Brian's oxygen saturations were low at 88%, Paul's mentor was correct to advise him not to increase the oxygen, but to give 2 litres/min via nasal cannulae while also giving an air-driven nebuliser via a face mask. Inpatients with COPD and the risk of hypercarbic respiratory failure should aim for oxygen saturations of 88–92% using only 24% oxygen via a venturi mask until ABG analysis is available (O'Driscoll et al., 2008). Brian's COPD was longstanding, and whereas hydrogen ions resulting from synthesis of carbon dioxide would normally be a major stimulus for breathing, people such as Brian, with long-term increased carbon dioxide levels, cease to respond to this stimulus. Instead, they depend on stimulation provided by a sensed reduction in oxygen levels (Porth, 1998). This means that had Paul increased Brian's oxygen to achieve normal oxygen saturation levels and Brian's chemoreceptors sensed adequate oxygen levels, the stimulus to breathe would be lost, causing Brian to have a respiratory arrest.

Brian's hypoxaemia required continued low-level oxygen therapy to correct it, but it was equally important to reduce his carbon dioxide level. Nebulising prescribed drugs such as salbutamol and ipratropium bromide to treat bronchoconstriction and reduce air trapping help to reduce the feeling of breathlessness and aid smoother air flow through the airways (Merritt, 2009). NICE (2010c) recommends increasing the frequency of nebulisers in exacerbations of COPD and to drive them with air in patients at risk of hypercarbic respiratory failure. Paul's mentor gave accurate instructions to Paul and observed guidelines that the nebuliser is ineffective once it starts to splutter (Boe et al., 2001).

Brian's inability to exhale sufficient carbon dioxide (CO_2 retention) was probably caused by sputum retention, although poor posture and air trapping could also contribute. Physiotherapy can help with clearing sputum by helping to shake it loose, precipitating coughing. Brian was able to do as the physiotherapist asked, cough and expectorate sputum, but had he been unable to do so, insertion of a naso-pharyngeal airway, through which secretions can be removed by suctioning, should be considered. Because Brian was already receiving antibiotic therapy for his exacerbation of COPD, it would be necessary to review their effectiveness in relation to available sputum culture results, which would indicate the antibiotic sensitivity.

Paul was quick to respond to Brian's respiratory distress by immediate ABCDE assessment using the 'Look: Listen: Feel: Measure' approach. He then acted upon his findings by asking for help, sitting Brian up, ensuring correct oxygen delivery, and continually monitoring Brian while he received nebuliser therapy. Paul's interventions under his mentor's guidance were instrumental in preventing deterioration that could have led to the need for NIV (Chapter 3) or respiratory arrest.

Monitoring to prevent breathlessness

Scenario: Asthma

You are working alongside the hospital respiratory nurse specialist and you are asked to gather initial information from patients as they arrive for asthma clinic appointments. You meet 24-year-old Liz Gardiner, who appears anxious, wheezy and a little out of breath. She tells you she has been rushing and that she will be fine in a few minutes.

Activity 2.5   *Critical thinking*

Make a list of the possible causes of Liz's symptoms and try to prioritise them in order of significance from very important to not important. Give reasons for your answer.

A list of symptoms and significance is given at the end of the chapter.

It is important that you observe Liz as she waits to see the respiratory nurse. She may be well enough to walk into the department and be convincing in her story, but she has an appointment time lasting only a few minutes and then she will leave again. You have very little time to determine whether or not Liz has health needs that require immediate attention by way of investigation, intervention or education. Anything that is not attended to now may have to wait six months, and during that time Liz may be at risk of severe respiratory problems leading to hypoxia and associated with uncontrolled asthma, infection or allergy. Any of these may require hospital admission.

Liz already has a diagnosis of asthma, a chronic inflammatory lung disorder that causes obstruction of airflow. The fact that she attends hospital appointments suggests that she has had problems in the past with control of her asthma or acute, life-threatening episodes (BTS and SIGN, 2009). Liz's breathlessness and wheeze on arrival are significant and warrant further exploration. After allowing her to rest for a few minutes, you should note her degree of recovery and inform the respiratory nurse. She will want to know what triggers Liz's wheeze and dyspnoea, the frequency that Liz has been experiencing symptoms such as breathlessness, wheeze, chest tightness or a cough, how she deals with them and how long they last (BTS and SIGN, 2009).

The respiratory nurse should review Liz's use of any asthma medication, such as inhalers for prevention or treatment of symptoms. She should check that Liz uses the correct techniques when using her inhalers, to ensure that medication is effectively administered. Any psychosocial factors that could contribute to exacerbating Liz's asthma should be considered, and it would be useful for Liz to use a peak flow meter to monitor and keep a diary of her peak expiratory flow rate (PEFR). Peak flow measurements give an indication of airway resistance by measuring the force of expiration in litres per minute (Wheeldon, 2009). Normal values of PEFR vary depending upon age, sex and height of the individual, and recordings of 70% of expected value or less indicate airway obstruction (BTS and SIGN, 2009). Peak flow trends are more useful than single values recorded, as they highlight deviations from normal for individual patients. These can serve to warn of potential instability in response to infection or other asthma triggers, thus allowing the patient to take appropriate preventative action. More information on peak flows can be obtained from the peak flow website listed at the end of the chapter.

Identifying the lowest level of treatment to maintain control for Liz's asthma and preventing life-threatening episodes depends upon her understanding her condition, being involved in monitoring and her honesty and concordance with prescribed therapy and health promotion advice. For this reason, the relationship that you develop with Liz on your first encounter could have implications for her lifelong respiratory health.

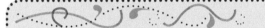

Chapter summary

Within this chapter we have used examples of patient situations to demonstrate why patients become breathless, how we can specifically assess breathing and the most appropriate interventions for some common clinical situations. We have considered patients in a variety of health care settings to demonstrate how acute situations can arise and how your response to acute situations can have significant impact upon patient outcomes.

Activities: brief outline answers

Activity 2.1: Critical thinking (page 29)

Table 2.3: Answer to Activity 2.1: different aspects of breathing that can be assessed

Assessment method	Making note of:	Significance
Look	Rate of breaths – how many per minute. Rhythm. Depth. Symmetry. Smoothness. Effort used.	Breathing should be effortless 10–20 breaths per minute. Bradypnoea (>10bpm) could be a sign of central nervous system depression. Tachypnoea (<20bpm) could indicate hypoxia but is normal after exercise. Both sides of chest should rise equally

Assessment method	Making note of:	Significance
	Facial expression – pursed lips, nasal flaring, grimace with pain. Use of accessory muscles. Ratio I:E (inspiration time: expiration time). General distress.	and evenly. Asymmetrical inflation could signify injury, pneumonectomy or pneumothorax. Mucous membranes should be pink and moist; pale mucous membranes could indicate low oxygen saturations or low haemoglobin content. Skin – should be pink and warm. Breathing should not be painful – pain could indicate infection of lungs, airways or inflammation of pleura. Distress, use of accessory muscles and facial expressions are evidence of hypoxia and need for patient to take bigger breaths.
Listen (with and without stethoscope)	Is breathing noisy or quiet? Where does the sound come from: throat, upper or lower airways? What type of sound? At what stage of the breath does the sound occur – inspiration or expiration? Beginning or end? Equality/symmetry. Front and back. Sound of each breath in and out. Airflow noise. Quality of breath sounds. Ability to speak – how many words?	Is normally quiet in clear airways and is quieter on expiration than inspiration. Different noises can indicate bronchospasm – (intermittent closing of the airways), blockage, sputum retention, pulmonary oedema. Visit http://solutions.3m.com/wps/portal/3M/en_US/3M-Littmann/stethoscope/littmann-learning-institute/ to listen to different breathing sounds. When using a stethoscope you will hear better quality sounds than without. Inability to complete sentences in one breath indicate hypoxia.
Feel	Breath/ air movement on hand. Chest expansion – rise and fall. Sensations on chest movement. Skin temperature. Movement.	Feeling for air movement can augment other methods of assessment to confirm what you see or hear, especially if breathing is shallow or you are in a noisy environment. Different sensations can indicate sputum retention (rattles), surgical emphysema (like crepe paper) or pulmonary oedema (boggy). Skin should be warm and dry to touch – cold clammy skin can indicate hypoxia.

Table 2.3: Continued

Continued

Assessment method	Making note of:	Significance
Measure	Number of breaths per minute. Size of breaths in millilitres. Force of breaths millilitres per second. Oxygen saturations. Acid base balance results from ABG analysis. Number of words spoken between breaths.	Respiratory Rate (RR), number of completes breaths (in and out) per minute, also known as respiration rate, respiratory frequency (Rf), Ventilation rate (VR), Ventilation frequency (Vf) breathing frequency (Bf) or pulmonary ventilation rate. These abbreviations may be seen on respiratory support equipment. The size in millilitres of a normal exhaled breath (without force) is known as (expiratory) tidal volume. This can only be effectively measured through a tracheostomy or endotracheal tube. Peak flow measures force of breaths and is useful to establish effects of therapy. Oxygen saturations in conjunction with therapy response: 98–100% in normal. 94–98% aim in acute. 88–92% in risk of HRF. Levels of oxygen in peripheral circulation and carbon dioxide in blood = type of respiratory failure. Gives an indication of degree of improvement or deterioration in breathing efficiency.

Table 2.3: Continued

Activity 2.3: Decision-making (page 32)

Sally French has more than one vital sign that falls outside normal ranges – her temperature, pulse rate and respiratory rate are high while her SaO_2 is low and her blood pressure is borderline low. She is currently receiving high flow oxygen via a non-rebreathing mask and her saturations are still low. This suggests that she will need further support and continued oxygen therapy and continual monitoring.

It is clear that the level 1 indicators apply to Sally, but as she is receiving single organ support (respiratory support) she really requires level 2 care and will need to be nursed in the High Dependency Unit.

Admission bundle   So far you have collected data relating to temperature, pulse, respirations, blood pressure and oxygen saturations, but you need to determine Sally's level of consciousness. Because your findings indicate that Sally is at high risk of deterioration, you will plan to monitor all of the above parameters continuously, and you will want your medical and nursing colleagues to be aware of these facts.

Recognition bundle   You will be constantly monitoring Sally and will have calculated her risk score in relation to your local track and trigger score. This will be high due to the fact that she has abnormalities in all categories. She has several indicators that should trigger consideration of sepsis (see Chapter 7), and you will want to tell the medical team about this.

Response bundle   Sally is at high risk of deterioration, so the critical care outreach team need to be contacted urgently. You will need to document and communicate your findings and concerns to them using the SBAR tool.

Activity 2.5: Critical thinking (page 39)

The possible reasons why Liz is anxious, wheezy and out of breath are given in order of importance.

1. She may have a chest infection: secretions and inflammation within the airways as a result of chest infection will narrow her airways and make Liz more prone to bronchospasm, which creates the wheeze. If the wheeze is audible without a stethoscope, it is significant. Wheeze indicates constriction of the airways, thus airflow is restricted and Liz will find it harder to breathe in the oxygen she needs, particularly if she is rushing and using more energy. This is the priority problem as it needs to be treated with antibiotics and Liz will need to temporarily increase the use of her inhalers, making sure that she takes both the preventer and reliever. She will also need to monitor her peak flows to make sure that her asthma symptoms are being adequately controlled. If Liz does not get early treatment for a chest infection, she could have severe respiratory difficulties, leading to hospitalisation and intensive care (BTS and SIGN, 2009).
2. Liz's asthma may not be as well controlled as she says it is. If she is getting anxious prior to her appointment and this is triggering wheeziness and shortness of breath, it is important to ascertain what Liz understands about her asthma symptoms and the medication she takes, how often she takes it, what time of day she takes it and her technique. She may need to increase her medication, she may need to be taught better inhaler techniques or she may not be taking her medication as prescribed. Liz may need some information to help her decision making. She may also need information about peak flow monitoring so that she can see clearly when her asthma is not well controlled. It would be useful to find out what triggers Liz's symptoms, and to reiterate when Liz needs to seek help from her doctor or respiratory nurse. Giving Liz good health promotion advice can help to prevent her asthma getting severely out of control and necessitating hospital admission.
3. Liz may have been subjected to an allergen that triggers her asthma symptoms while on her journey. Much of the educational and health promotion information detailed in Answer 2 still applies as it is important that Liz responds quickly when her asthma is triggered.
4. She may just have been rushing, and may have had a stressful journey. However, she is clearly showing symptoms of asthma, which should ideally be better controlled. Good health promotion advice is needed as in Answer 2.

Further reading

Higginson, R and Jones, B (2009) Respiratory assessment in critically ill patients: airway and breathing. *British Journal of Nursing*, 18(8): 456–61.

This article gives a good overview of respiratory assessment and the skills needed by ward nurses as well as critical care nurses. There is clear advice about use of oxygen masks.

O'Driscoll, B R, Howard, L S and Davison, A G (2008) *Guidelines for emergency oxygen use in adult patients: executive summary*. London: British Thoracic Society.

These are the guidelines for oxygen use that should be applied nationally. This is information that all nurses need to know.

Robinson, T and Scullion, J E (2009) *Oxford handbook of respiratory nursing*. Oxford: Oxford University Press.

This book is a pocket-sized resource giving practical advice and current best practice for a range of respiratory conditions.

Useful websites

www.lunguk.org/

The British Lung Foundation website has information about most lung conditions, including pneumonia and COPD.

http://solutions.3m.com/wps/portal/3M/en_US/3M-Littmann/stethoscope/littmann-learning-institute/

The 3M™ Littman® Stethoscopes website offers informative advice about the use and care of stethoscopes as well as having audio clips of heart and lung sounds.

www.peakflow.com/top_nav/normal_values/PEFNorms.html

The Mini-Wright Peak Flow Meter site offers clear information about peak flow monitoring and devices used. There is patient information as well as professional information and links to other useful organisations.

www.asthma.org.uk/index.html

The Asthma UK website gives a lot of information about asthma including inhalers and nebulisers. There is information that is useful for professionals and patients alike.

Chapter 3
The patient who needs respiratory support

Desiree Tait

Introduction

Scenario: John Paul's story

John Paul is a third-year student nurse who agreed to work two night shifts with his mentor in order to gain an understanding of 24-hour care provision in the intensive care unit (ICU). He was looking forward to a quiet night when they had a phone call from a staff nurse on the medical ward that had a patient with a high risk trigger score. Using the SBAR tool (see Chapter 1, Table 1.8) she presented the following information over the telephone.

- Patient name and age*: Gladys Cabrera, age 63 years, African Caribbean.*
- Situation*: I am concerned about this lady who was admitted 12 hours ago at 11.00 hours with an acute exacerbation of chronic obstructive pulmonary disease (COPD). She has become increasingly breathless and tired. The 24% O_2 and nebuliser therapy did not improve her condition and the medical team have commenced an **aminophylline** infusion but there is still no improvement.*
- Background*: Gladys has a seven-year history of acute exacerbations of COPD and has been admitted to hospital twice in the last three years for this condition. On this admission she has undergone sepsis screening, blood cultures have been collected and she is on broad spectrum antibiotic therapy. A chest X-ray has confirmed evidence of consolidation in both lungs.*
- Assessment*: She is unable to talk due to her breathlessness, she is sitting upright in bed, and, using her accessory respiratory muscles, her breathing is noisy and she appears centrally cyanosed with blue mucous membranes. She is hot and agitated but able to respond to commands, T: 38.5°C, R: 40/min, P: 180, BP: 180/90, SaO_2: 72%, track and trigger score has increased from 5 to 8 in the last 30 minutes, and the house officer is on his way to ICU with her arterial blood sample for analysis.*
- Recommendation*: I am concerned that Gladys's condition is now critical and she needs an urgent assessment.*

The results of Gladys's arterial sample are:

pH: 7.29
PaO_2: 4.8 kPa
$PaCO_2$: 8.4 kPa
HCO_3: 28.5 mmol/l
BE (base excess) +7

John Paul's mentor asks the nurse on the ward to increase the air flow of the 24% oxygen mask to 6l/min and to stay with the patient – the outreach team will be there in 3–5 minutes. In the meantime a bed is prepared in ICU.

Following a rapid assessment of Gladys's condition, it was agreed that an escalation of treatment was required (NICE 2010c). Gladys's respiratory problems have required her to be admitted to hospital before, but up until now these have always been managed by the medical team in acute care. She is too breathless to ask questions, so the staff try to explain what is happening and why. Gladys will need advanced respiratory support with non-invasive ventilation in order to resolve type II respiratory failure and an increase in the percentage of oxygen therapy to resolve the hypoxaemia (see Chapter 2). John Paul holds Gladys's hand, not sure what to do next, and the ward nurse goes to phone the relatives to inform them of the change in Gladys's condition and location.

Why did Gladys require an escalation of treatment?

Using 'Look: Listen: Feel: Measure', we can see that the management regime has failed to improve her condition (NICE, 2010c). Gladys was using her accessory muscles to breathe and could not verbalise because of her shortness of breath. The ward nurse assumed the presence of cyanosis, but Gladys is African Caribbean and there is evidence to suggest that some people can have a slightly blue tinge to their lips when healthy due to high levels of pigmentation, so it is therefore important to assess inside her mouth and tongue as well as monitoring her SaO_2 (Bickley, 2008). For Gladys, an SaO_2 of 72% in the presence of assumed central cyanosis indicated that she was suffering from severe hypoxia and was critically ill. Increased respiratory rate, heart rate and blood pressure are indications that she is using all her physiological resources to keep breathing and if she continues to exert this amount of effort for much longer, she could suffer a hypoxia-induced cardiac arrest. A rapid and comprehensive assessment is essential, accompanied by an escalation of treatment (O'Driscoll et al., 2008). These findings are reinforced by the arterial blood gas results, which indicate evidence of acidosis (pH 7.29), and type II respiratory failure (PaO_2: 4.8kPa, $PaCO_2$: 8.4kPa) as discussed in Chapter 2. Patients with COPD and type II respiratory failure have an increased sensitivity to changes in oxygen levels, so in Gladys's case it was appropriate to ask the nurse on the ward to increase the rate of flow through the mask, thus increasing the flow pressure rather than the concentration of oxygen until the outreach team arrived minutes later (O'Driscoll et al., 2008).

Why are the arterial blood gas results significant?

In the body, acids (substances that release hydrogen ions (H^+) in solution) are constantly being produced as by-products of normal cell metabolism. For example, the metabolism of proteins produces acids such as sulphuric acid and hydrochloric acid. During the metabolism of carbohydrates 15,000mmol of carbon dioxide (CO_2) is produced each day, and although it is not an acid, it is influential in maintaining pH balance. Carbon dioxide is transported in the circulation in the following ways.

* Attached to haemoglobin and carried as carbaminohaemoglobin ($HbCO_2$, 20%) and exhaled from the lungs as CO_2 and H_2O.
* Dissolved in the plasma (10%).
* As a bicarbonate base: a substance that uses up hydrogen ions (70%).

Left in the circulation, an imbalance in acids or bases would destroy cells and organs, so it is imperative the body has ways to maintain a pH balance at a pH value of between 7.35 and 7.45 in order to maintain normal cell function (Hall, 2011). Should the pH value fall above or below this range the impact on the body can be critical and in extreme cases lead to death. The results obtained from analysis of arterial blood provides information about a number of factors involved in the process of acid-base balance as well as information about the amount of oxygen available to the cells. These include:

* pH value;
* the amount of O_2 in the blood (expressed as the partial pressure of oxygen or PaO_2);
* the amount of CO_2 in the blood (expressed as the partial pressure of carbon dioxide or $PaCO_2$);
* the amount of bicarbonate and bases available to buffer acids (expressed as mmol/l);
* potassium;
* haemoglobin;
* urea and creatinine.

Why are these values important?

The body has a number of ways of maintaining the acid-base balance in health and we will look at three now.

Buffer systems are control mechanisms that can either increase or decrease the number of hydrogen ions in a solution, thus making the solution more acid if the hydrogen ions increase in number or more alkaline if the hydrogen ions are reduced in number (Mattson Porth and Matfin, 2009). These include:

* protein buffer systems such as the plasma proteins;
* bicarbonate buffer system that converts a strong acid that releases large numbers of H^+ to a weak acid that releases much fewer H^+. For example, hydrochloric acid (HCL: strong acid) can be substituted by carbonic acid (H_2CO_3: weak acid), thus reducing the overall H^+:

$$HCl + NaHCO_3 \rightleftharpoons H_2CO_3 + NaCl$$
$$\text{(sodium bicarbonate)} \qquad\qquad \text{(sodium chloride)}$$

This equation is reversible and is accelerated by the presence of the enzyme carbonic anhydrase. The carbonic acid produced dissociates into H^+ and HCO_3^- (bicarbonate ions). The H^+ combines with haemoglobin and the bicarbonate diffuses into plasma where it continues to participate in buffering acids;

* hydrogen-potassium exchange: when there is excess H^+ in the blood, some is able to move into cells in exchange for potassium ions (K^+), and when there is excess K^+ in the blood, it

moves into cells and exchanges with H^+. Thus potassium levels and hydrogen levels can change dramatically in some clinical situations such as a patient with diabetic ketoacidosis where potassium levels will be influenced by both levels of insulin and a metabolic acidosis.

Respiratory control mechanisms act as another line of defence against alterations in acid-base balance. An increase in ventilation decreases levels of CO_2, and a decrease in ventilation increases CO_2 in the blood. Chemo receptors in the brain stem, carotid and aortic bodies (see Figure 6.1, p114) sense changes in CO_2, H^+ and O_2 and alter the respiratory rate accordingly. The respiratory control of pH is rapid and occurs within minutes of a change in pH balance but is only approximately 50–70% effective as a buffer system. It is the first line of defence against large changes in pH.

Renal control mechanisms are slow to react but can continue to function for days until the pH value has returned to the normal range. The mechanisms are:

* reabsorption of bicarbonate ions into the circulation;
* excretion of hydrogen ions from acids produced as a result of protein and fat metabolism.

What do these values tell us?

The pH value determines the presence of acidaemia and alkalaemia.

* acidaemia: pH <7.35
* alkalaemia: pH <7.45

The partial pressures of oxygen and carbon dioxide give a measure of respiratory function and the presence of respiratory acidosis/alkalosis.

* Respiratory acidosis:
    * pH <7.35 and $PaCO_2$ >6.0 kPa;
    * dyspnoea/increased or decreased respiratory function;
    * headache;
    * restlessness, confusion;
    * drowsiness/unconsciousness;
    * tachycardia and arrhythmias.
* Respiratory alkalosis:
    * pH>7.45 and $PaCO_2$< 4.9kPa;
    * feeling light-headed;
    * numbness and tingling in the mouth and peripheries;
    * inability to concentrate, confusion;
    * palpitations.

The levels of bicarbonate and base excess give a measure of metabolic function and represent either a failure to buffer hydrogen ion concentrations with bases leading to acidosis or a failure to buffer bicarbonate concentrations with acids leading to an alkalosis.

* Metabolic acidosis:
    * pH<7.35 and HCO_3 <22 mmol/L;
    * headache;
    * restlessness, confusion;
    * coma;

- cardiac arrhythmias;
- Kussmaul respirations (rapid shallow)/respiratory depression;
- skin warm and flushed.
- Metabolic alkalosis:
  - pH >7.45 and HCO_3 >27mmol/L;
  - muscle twitching and cramps;
  - feeling dizzy;
  - confusion;
  - lethargy;
  - seizures/coma;
  - nausea and vomiting.

In Table 3.1 you will find clinical examples of patients who have experienced an acid-base imbalance.

Arterial blood gas analysis	Patient examples
Respiratory acidosis: pH <7.35 $PaCO_2$ >6.0kPa	See Gladys Cabrera's story (pages 46–7)
Respiratory alkalosis: pH >7.45 $PaCO_2$ <4.9kPa	Joan Baker (50 years) suffers from anxiety attacks, and these have become worse since progressing to the menopause. On this occassion she has been involved in a minor road traffic collision and she has no obvious injuries. However, when the paramedics arrived at the scene they found her to be breathless and disorientated. She was complaining of pins and needles in her hands and arms, and she felt she couldn't get her breath. Joan was taken to accident and emergency where her arterial blood gas result following admission was: pH: 7.49; $PaCO_2$: 3.2kPa; HCO_3: 24.2mmols/l; BE: −1.0. Joan was hyperventilating and needed to be encouraged to reduce her respiratory rate and allow her carbon dioxide levels to rise back to normal levels.
Metabolic acidosis: pH <7.35 HCO_3 <22mmol/l	Mary Bevan (58 years) was found by her neighbour lying at the front door in a drowsy and confused state. Mary has type 2 diabetes and has recently developed a severe infection on her leg. Mary's neighbour called the emergency services and Mary was admitted to accident and emergency. Her arterial blood gas following admission was: pH: 7.24; $PaCO_2$: 3.8kPa; HCO_3: 15.1 mmols/l; BE: −13.7. Mary had Kussmaul respirations at a rate of 35/min and a blood glucose of 22mmol/l. Mary had developed a metabolic acidosis secondary to infection that triggered an increase in blood glucose that necessitated management with insulin.

Table 3.1: Clinical examples of patients with changes in acid-base balance

Arterial blood gas analysis	Patient examples
Metabolic alkalosis: pH >7.45 HCO$_3$ >26mmol/L	Gary Smith (54 years) has been suffering from indigestion-type pain for several days. Rather than go to the GP he has been treating himself with large doses of antacids such as bicarbonate of soda. That afternoon he felt nauseated, weak and tired and still had the persistent indigestion. He visited the GP who decided to admit him to hospital for an assessment of his chest pain. His arterial blood gas following admission was: pH: 7.49; PaCO$_2$: 5.6kPa; HCO$_3$: 29.7mmol/l; BEs: +9.0.
Respiratory and metabolic acidosis pH <7.35 PaCO$_2$ >6.0kPa HCO$_3$ <22mmol/l	Peter Baker (41 years) was admitted to an acute ward with a history of abdominal pain, nausea and vomiting. Peter's condition deteriorated during the first 24 hours, and that evening he had a cardiac arrest. He was resuscitated and transfered to ICU for respiratory support and management of acute pancreatitis. His arterial blood gas following admission was: pH: 7.15; PaCO$_2$: 7.6kPa; HCO$_3$: 16.7mmol/l; BEs: –9.8. Peter has developed a combined acidosis as a result of his cardiac arrest (failed respiration) and severe sepsis associated with pancreatitis (see Chapter 7).

Table 3.1: Continued

What are the implications of the arterial blood gas results for Gladys?

If we analyse Gladys's arterial blood sample and her general condition, we can see that she meets the criteria for NIV (RCP, BTS and ICS, 2008).

- pH 7.29 and PaCO$_2$ 8.4kPa show evidence of respiratory acidosis; she is also dyspnoeic, hot and agitated with a tachycardia of 180/min.
- PaO$_2$: 4.8 kPa shows evidence of hypoxaemia.
- HCO$_3$: 28.5 mmol/l and BE (base excess) +7 shows evidence that Gladys's kidneys have been compensating for an abnormally high CO$_2$ because of COPD. However, during this acute exacerbation of COPD her lungs are unable to cope because of the respiratory infection. As a result, her oxygen levels are falling and her carbon dioxide levels are increasing. This means that her respiratory system is no longer able to prevent life-threatening hypoxia and control her acid-base balance without extra respiratory support. A step-by-step guide to arterial blood gas analysis is summarised in Table 3.2.

Always risk assess	Look: Listen: Feel: Measure
ABG: Step 1 Assess oxygenation. Normal: PaO_2 11.5–13.5kPa	Is there evidence of hypoxaemia? Is there evidence of high levels of oxygenation? Is the patient receiving supplemental oxygen?
ABG: Step 2 Assess pH level. Normal: 7.35–7.45	Is there evidence of acidosis? pH <7.35 Is there evidence of alkalosis? pH >7.45
ABG: Step 3 Assess the respiratory component. $PaCO_2$: 4.5–6.0kPa	Is the $PaCO_2$ <4.5kPa? Is the $PaCO_2$ >6.0 kPa?
ABG: Step 4 Assess the metabolic component. HCO_3^-: 22–27 mmol/l	Is the HCO_3^- <22 mmol/l? Is the HCO_3^- >27 mmol/l? The base excess level (BE) is the quantity of acid or base required to restore the pH to 7.4. Base excess will mirror the bicarbonate level and simply reinforces evidence of a metabolic component (Jevon and Ewens, 2007).
ABG: Step 5	Combine your findings from steps 2/3/4 and identify if there is evidence of: • respiratory acidosis; • respiratory alkalosis; • metabolic acidosis; • metabolic alkalosis; • signs that the respiratory system have compensated for a metabolic acidosis by increasing the respiratory rate and reducing the CO_2 level; • signs that the renal system have compensated for chronic respiratory acidosis by increasing the level of HCO_3.
ABG: Step 6	Interpret the ABGs in the context of all available patient data.

Table 3.2: A step-by-step approach to assessing arterial blood gas results (ABG)

Activity 3.1   *Decision-making*

Read the scenario below and think about the significance of the arterial blood gas results.

Joseph Baglio (age 68 years) has smoked 40 cigarettes a day since his twenties and was admitted to the medical ward six hours ago following a diagnosis of pneumonia. Unfortunately, Joseph deteriorated suddenly; his chest was noisy and he was finding it

continued . . .

difficult to breathe. He had a cardiac arrest ten minutes later. Joe was resuscitated successfully. His arterial blood gas results 30 minutes after his resuscitation were:

pH: 7.07
PaO_2: 8.5kPa
$PaCO_2$: 14.1kPa
HCO_3: 22.5mmol/l
BE: −3.0

Joseph was conscious, flushed and anxious. His vital signs were T: 38.0°C, R: 30/min, P: 95, BP: 130/85mmHg. He was receiving 60% oxygen.

* Using the step-by-step guide in Table 3.2, what can you interpret from the arterial blood gas result?
* What are your priorities of care for this patient?

Joseph was reviewed four hours later and his arterial blood gas results were:

pH: 7.30
PaO_2: 10.4kPa
$PaCO_2$: 6.70kPa
HCO_3: 25.7mmol/l
BE: +1.3

Joseph was conscious but tired. His vital signs were T: 38.0°C, R: 25/min, P: 90, BP: 120/80mmHg. He was receiving 60% oxygen.

* Using the step-by-step guide in Table 3.2, what can you interpret from the arterial blood gas result?
* What are your priorities of care for this patient?

Answers are given at the end of the chapter.

Gladys has type II respiratory failure and is on her way to ICU. The next case study describes Gladys's own perspective of her arrival on the unit.

Case study: Gladys arrives in ICU

When Gladys arrived in ICU she felt very tired; it was getting harder to breathe and she kept forgetting where she was and what the nurses were telling her. They gave her a funny-looking oxygen mask to hold and asked her to hold it close to her face so that she could get used to it. She didn't like it – her face felt as though it was standing in front of a wind machine – but the young lad who came to see her on the ward kept holding her hand and reassured her that it would help her to feel better. After a few minutes they tied the mask to her face and she got the full force of air rushing in. It felt very tight on her face and head but she did feel as though she was getting more air now. 'Perhaps I'll be able to rest soon,' she thought. The young lad was still holding her hand and people were doing something with her wrist. It was stinging – something about an artery and gases. 'I wonder if Stanley knows I'm here. Oh yes, that young lad (what is his name?) said he would be in to see me later. I want to pull this mask off,' she thought. 'I'll just try . . .'

What is NIV and why is it appropriate to use this respiratory support for Gladys?

Pulmonary ventilation or breathing is essential for life, and the purpose of NIV is to provide varying levels of positive pressure air flow through a tight-fitting mask in order to improve the patient's levels of PaO_2 and $PACO_2$. Breathing involves the inhalation of gases in air into the lungs and exhalation of gases from the lungs into the atmosphere. All gases in air collectively exert a pressure known as atmospheric pressure. The gases in the lungs also exert a pressure known as alveolar pressure. In air, gases always flow from an area of high pressure to an area of low pressure. During inspiration the thoracic space expands as a result of contraction of the intercostal muscles and diaphragm. This increase in space reduces the overall alveolar pressure in the lungs, and air flows into the airways in order to equalise the pressure. Expiration involves relaxation of the respiratory muscles and natural elastic recoil of the lung tissue so that air flows back into the atmosphere. Normal breathing therefore relies on negative pressure ventilation.

For 120 years the principal method of supporting ventilation for patients with respiratory failure was based on the principle of negative pressure ventilation. For example, the **iron lung** was used successfully for patients with respiratory failure caused by neuromuscular diseases such as polio. In the 1950s during the polio epidemic in Europe the demand for iron lungs outstripped supply, and alternative methods for providing respiratory support were attempted (Lassen et al., 1954). This led to the development of mechanical **invasive ventilation**, which involved air being forced under pressure into patients' lungs via a tracheostomy tube or endotracheal tube at a rate of between 10 and 20 per minute in order to mimic normal respiration. This dramatically reduced the mortality rate of patients suffering from respiratory failure and became the mainstay treatment.

In the last 25 years the use of positive pressure non-invasive ventilation (NIV) techniques that supply air through a tight-fitting face mask rather than a tube have escalated, and this method has now become the first-line therapy for adult patients with:

- sleep apnoea;
- acute exacerbations of COPD;
- pulmonary oedema;
- neuromuscular disease;
- pneumonia;
- weaning from MIV.

The types of NIV and their use are explained in Table 3.3.

Activity 3.2 — *Reflection*

Reflect back on patients you have nursed and ask yourself the following questions.

- Have I looked after patients with acute respiratory failure either in hospital or the community?
- If so, how did I assess and document the patient care?
- Did the patient need support with oxygen therapy or NIV?
- Did the patient have support from the physiotherapist, dietitian and respiratory nurse?

Hint: This reflection is meant to encourage you to think critically about assessing and managing care and should help you to identify good practice and areas for improvement.

As this answer is based on your own reflection, there is no outline answer at the end of the chapter.

Type of NIV	Benefits	Risks	Patient examples
Continuous positive airways pressure: *CPAP.* This method provides a continuous flow of positive pressure even at the end of expiration so that some air always remains trapped in the alveoli. This enables oxygen exchange to continue during the whole respiratory cycle and prevents alveolar collapse (atelactasis).	• Improves oxygenation in patients with type I respiratory failure. • Reduces the risk of atelactasis.	• There is reduced clearance of CO_2 due to air being trapped in the alveoli. Not suitable for patients with type II respiratory failure where there is increased levels of CO_2. • The airway is not protected so patients must be able to maintain their own airway.	• Mrs Smith is admitted with severe breathlessness and is producing excessive amounts of pink frothy secretions from her airways. She is diagnosed with acute pulmonary oedema and is commenced on CPAP starting at 5cm H_2O as part of her ongoing treatment to reduce pulmonary secretions by increasing alveolar pressure to above capillary hydrostatic pressure. • Chao Chan is diagnosed with pneumonia and type I respiratory failure. His PaO_2 is 6.2kPa and his $PaCO_2$ is 3.6kPa. He is commenced on CPAP at 5 and then 10cm H_2O. • Bryn Jones has been diagnosed with **obstructive sleep apnoea.** He suffers from morbid obesity, snoring and daytime fatigue. He has now been fitted with a face mask and CPAP machine for home use. The equipment delivers CPAP at 10cm H_2O, to be used at night while sleeping

Table 3.3: Types of non-invasive ventilation and their use

Continued

Type of NIV	Benefits	Risks	Patient examples
Bilevel NIV or bilevel positive airways pressure ventilation: *BiPAP*. This method provides two alternating levels of positive pressure during respiration. During inspiration there is an inspired pressure level IPAP and during expiration, an expired pressure level: EPAP.	• Improves oxygenation and CO_2 clearance in patients with type II respiratory failure • IPAP reduces the work of breathing and conserves the use of oxygen by the body. • A lower EPAP pressure reduces air trapping but still allows continuous gas exchange during respiration while preventing atelactasis.	• The airway is not protected so patients must be able to maintain their own airway.	• Gladys Cabrera as illustrated in the case study. • Henry Jones has pneumonia. His PaO_2 is 6.8kPa and his $PaCO_2$ is 6.5kPa. He is breathless and agitated. He is commenced on BiPAP with an inspiratory pressure of 10cm H_2O and an expiratory pressure of 4 cm H_2O.

Table 3.3: Continued

Contraindications for using NIV

The success of NIV techniques in the support of respiratory function rely on effective patient selection. For Gladys, BiPAP is the optimum treatment regime, but this does not mean that the use of NIV will always lead to a successful outcome for every patient. Patients need to be risk assessed for any contraindications before commencing the therapy and then risk assessed for evidence of any change or deterioration in their condition. This is illustrated in Table 3.4. The contraindications listed below rarely exist in isolation: often patients will present with one or more of these factors. Knowing the patient and their medical history is an essential part of the rapid decision-making process required when determining a patient's suitability for NIV and relies on good communication between all the carers involved (RCP et al., 2008). Contraindications include:

- life-threatening hypoxaemia;
- severe confusion/agitation/cognitive impairment;
- unconscious patient;
- airway obstruction due to vomiting or a foreign object;
- facial trauma/burns/surgery;
- undrained **pneumothorax**;
- patient unable to protect their own airway;
- copious amounts of respiratory secretions/sputum;
- recent surgery in the upper gastro-intestinal tract;
- severe co-morbidity;
- haemodynamic instability;
- presence of bowel obstruction.

Risk assessment	Nursing interventions
Contraindications for use of NIV	• Rapid assessment of ABCDE using 'Look: Listen: Feel: Measure' is important to measure the risk of contraindications to treatment with NIV. In particular, the risk of pneumothorax should be ruled out by reviewing the patient's chest X-ray following their admission. • A patient may decide to refuse treatment.
Preparation of the patient and technology	• If the patient has consented and is able to proceed, ensure the equipment has been prepared and checked to ensure it is in working order. • Sit the patient upright and, with their cooperation, attach the face mask. The patient will need a few minutes to get used to the mask. Often NIV is commenced at a low level and increased according to the clinical state of the patient (RCP et al., 2008). • Document base-line clinical data. • Agree and document a treatment plan for escalating and identifying a ceiling of treatment.

Table 3.4: Risk assessment and management of patients receiving NIV

Continued

Risk assessment	Nursing interventions

Airway and respirations	• Monitor the patient's airway and respiratory rate, look for signs of respiratory distress and air entry as illustrated in Figure 2.1, p30.
	• Monitor SaO_2 for evidence of improvement or deterioration.
	• Monitor the patient's arterial blood gas results after:
	  • one hour: if there is no change in the patient's condition or a slight improvement, then monitor again in four hours.
	  • one hour: if there is a deterioration in the patient's condition:
	    • assess patient and check the equipment;
	    • consider either increasing the oxygen or pressures;
	    • consider a change to mechanical ventilation.

Haemodynamic state	• The increase in pulmonary airway pressure from NIV can cause a rebound reduction in the patient's blood pressure, particularly with CPAP pressures above 10cm H_2O. • Monitor the patient's blood pressure every five minutes during the first 30 minutes and then at 30 minutes to hourly as the patient's blood pressure stabilises. Continuous arterial monitoring of blood pressure provides an effective way to monitor BP as well as obtaining arterial samples for blood gas analysis.
Mental state and level of consciousness	• Monitor for signs of increased confusion or agitation. Any deterioration in level of consciousness is an indication that the NIV should be discontinued and the treatment plan utilised. • Patients on NIV should not be sedated as this can compromise their airway and compliance with treatment.
Fluid balance and gastro-intestinal function	• There is a risk of fluid retention triggered by the stress response (Chapter 6). Look for evidence of reduced urine output and interstitial oedema. • There is a risk of increased air swallowing and gastric distension associated with the air flow. This may be reduced by inserting a nasogastric tube.
Psychological distress	• Patients receiving NIV experience discomfort and distress due to the tight-fitting mask and side effects of the treatment. Communication is difficult with the face mask in place, although this may be resolved for some patients by using a nasal mask. Alternative techniques for delivering the air under pressure include a mouth piece and a helmet. • The role of the nurse in providing support and reassurance is essential. Frequent removal of the mask is counterproductive, and it is important to encourage the patient to keep the mask in situ for at least 30 minutes if any benifit is to be achieved. • If a patient is becoming very distressed, this will impact on their physiological state and is often an indication to discontinue the NIV and refer to the treatment plan (Jarvis, 2006). • Optimum management of patients with acute respiratory failure and NIV is achieved in ICU. However, patients can be nursed in acute wards and accident and emergency provided there is an appropriate skill mix and staff ratios of 1 or 2 patients: 1 nurse.

Table 3.4: Continued

Case study: Gladys Cabrera

Gladys was commenced on BiPAP at an inspiration pressure (IPAP) of 12cm H_2O and an expired pressure (EPAP) of 5cm H_2O with 40% oxygen. She didn't like the face mask but was prepared to give it a try as long as the nurse reminded her. An hour later, 00:30 hours, her vital signs were: T: 38.0°C, R: 35/min, P: 140, BP: 120/80, SaO_2: 86%. Arterial blood gases revealed an improvement in her oxygenation and carbon dioxide levels although there was still some evidence of acidaemia:

pH: 7.32
PaO_2: 8.8kPa
$PaCO_2$: 7.4kPa
HCO_3: 28.6mmol/l
BE: +8

Gladys appeared to be calmer but was complaining of a dry mouth and sore cheeks from the mask. The nurse repositioned the face mask so that the pressure was relieved and reassured her that the mask, while uncomfortable, was helping her breathing. Gladys was given sips of water to moisten her mouth. The treatment plan at this stage was to continue with the current respiratory support for a further four hours and review. If there were signs of deterioration in her respiratory rate, level of consciousness and/or her levels of SaO_2, then the team would escalate treatment to mechanical invasive respiratory support.

Four hours later (04:30 hours) Gladys was tired but feeling more comfortable. Her vital signs were T: 37.5°C, R: 28/min, P: 120, BP: 120/80, SaO_2: 90%. Arterial blood gases again revealed an improvement in her oxygenation and carbon dioxide levels:

pH: 7.35
PaO_2: 10.8kPa
$PaCO_2$: 7.0kPa
HCO_3: 28.5mmol/l
BE: +7

The plan was to reduce the oxygen concentration to 24% and continue with the NIV for a further four hours. Should Gladys continue to improve, the plan was to discontinue the NIV in the morning and manage Gladys's respiratory problem with the aid of physiotherapy, **prednisilone**, nebulised short-acting **beta agonist**, short acting **muscarinic antagonist** and intravenous antibiotics. By 09:00 hours the next morning her vital signs were: T: 37.0°C, R: 26/min, P: 100, BP: 120/76, SaO_2: 92%. Arterial blood gases again revealed an improvement in her oxygenation and carbon dioxide levels:

pH: 7.35
PaO_2: 10.9kPa
$PaCO_2$: 6.8kPa
HCO_3: 28.6mmol/l
BE: +8

Gladys was discharged back to the ward the following afternoon and discharged home five days later under the care of the chronic conditions team and her general practitioner. Gladys's story is an example of how rapid assessment of a patient, collaboration between the patient and members of the health care team and patient-focused care can produce a positive patient outcome.

What happens when NIV is not suitable: the case for mechanical invasive ventilation (MIV)

The benefits of supporting patients with respiratory failure with NIV include the following (RCP et al., 2008).

*   There is reduced risk of ventilator-acquired pneumonia.
*   The patient is fully awake and an active partner in their care.
*   The patient may be nursed in an acute care setting.
*   The use of NIV may prevent the requirement for invasive respiratory support.

There are, however, a number of reasons why patients may require an escalation of treatment to MIV or direct intervention with MIV without NIV (Brainard and Deutschman, 2010). These include:

*   life-threatening hypoxic (PaO_2 below 8.0kPa) respiratory failure accompanied by patient confusion and/or exhaustion;
*   life-threatening hypercarbic ($PaCO_2$ above 6.0kPa) respiratory failure accompanied by patient confusion and/or exhaustion;
*   impaired consciousness and/or the patient's inability to protect their airway.

For patients in these situations, clinical assessment, combined with medical and nursing experience, is the most important tool for judging when invasive support with intubation and mechanical ventilation are required. Some clinical examples of these situations are included in Table 3.5 and explored in the case study of Billy Brown.

Case study: Introducing Billy Brown

*Billy Brown is 29 years old. He is homeless and for the last four weeks has been squatting in a derelict building on the edge of an industrial estate. Billy has been drinking up to 16 cans of lager a day since he was 11, when he can; he smokes 15 cigarettes a day and takes recreational drugs. He is unemployed but is ever hopeful of finding work and a permanent address. Billy was drinking with his mates in a local park one afternoon when they were asked to leave by the police. As Billy started to make a move he collapsed on the grass complaining of severe abdominal pain. He was admitted to the acute surgical unit and diagnosed with **acute pancreatitis**. Two days later Billy's condition deteriorated. On assessment ('Look: Listen: Feel: Measure') he was:*

> *breathless; confused and agitated; hot*
> *T: 38°C, R: 30/min, P: 98/min, BP: 110/60mmHg and SaO_2: 94%*

Billy's patient at risk score was within the acceptable range, but the nurse was concerned about his breathlessness and contacted the senior house officer.

Reason for MIV	Look: Listen: Feel: Measure	Patient examples
Hypoxaemic respiratory failure. • Pneumonia. • Lung consolidation. • Atelactasis. • Pulmonary oedema. • Acute respiratory distress syndrome (ARDS). • **Pulmonary embolism.** • **Carbon monoxide poisoning.**	Central cyanosis. Altered respiratory pattern. Agitation/irritability. Confusion. Exhaustion. Seizures. SaO_2 <85%. PaO_2 <8.0kPa.	Chao Chan (Table 3.3) is diagnosed with pneumonia and type I respiratory failure. His PaO_2 is 6.2kPa and his $PaCO_2$ is 3.6kPa. He was commenced on CPAP at 5cm H_2O then 10 cm H_2O. However, after the first hour he was confused and agitated, pulling off his mask and refusing to put it back on. His ABGs were PaO_2 5.7kPa and $PaCO_2$ 5.0kPa. It was agreed that treatment should be escalated to MIV.
Hypercarbic respiratory failure. • COPD. • Asthma. • Airway obstruction/ anatomical deformity. • Cervical injury above level C4 and/or damage to the brain stem. • Excessive sedation. • **Guillain-Barré Syndrome.** • Cardiac arrest. • Heart failure. • Pulmonary embolism.	Increased work of breathing. Use of accessory muscles. Shallow breathing. **Dyspnoea.** Agitation/irritability. Confusion. Exhaustion. Seizures. Cardiovascular collapse and cardiac arrest. $PaCO_2$ >6.0kPa.	Mariana Banica (27 years) has a severe scoliosis of her spine (the spine is curved from side to side in an S shape). Since childhood she has been prone to respiratory infections due to reduced and uneven lung capacity. Mariana was admitted to ICU after having collapsed at home following a flu-like illness for three days. On admission she was very confused, cyanosed and her breathing was shallow. Her ABGs were: pH: 7.19; PaO_2: 12.7kPa; $PaCO_2$: 10.7kPa; HCO_3: 24.0mmols/l; BE: 0.1. Mariana was intubated and commenced on bilevel positive pressure ventilation at a rate of 15/min, with an IPAP of 20cm H_2O and EPAP of 5cm H_2O.

Table 3.5: Indications for mechanical invasive ventilation in the critically ill patient

Reason for MIV	Look: Listen: Feel: Measure	Patient examples
Impaired consciousness and/or the patient's inability to protect his/her airway. • Glasgow Coma Scale (GCS) score of <8 indicates the potential for further deterioration in consciousness, reduced ventilation and poor airway protection. For example: • severe brain injury; • prolonged effects of general anaesthetic; • traumatic injury of the face and neck.	Inability to maintain airway. Unconscious. GCS <8.	Pete Williams (19 years) was assaulted on his way home from the pub. A witness said that Pete had been kicked repeatedly on the head while he lay on the floor. In ICU he was agitated and unable to communicate except with grunts. He was opening his eyes and flexing his arms to pain, GCS 7. The computerised tomography scan showed evidence of progressive brain swelling. The management plan for Pete in the first 24 hours was to intubate him with an oral endotracheal tube and provide continuous pressure ventilation (IPAP 30cm H_2O) with a rate of 15/min in order to protect his airway and maintain PaO_2 >8.0kPa and $PaCO_2$ 4.5–6.0kPa. Pete developed ventilator-acquired pneumonia on day four and stayed on MIV for seven days.

Table 3.5: Continued

Billy had already been screened for sepsis and commenced on antibiotic therapy. However, the house officer was concerned that he might have developed respiratory failure secondary to acute pancreatitis and sepsis. An arterial blood gas (ABG) sample confirmed his concerns:

pH: 7.36
PaO_2: 7.9kPa
$PaCO_2$: 4.9kPa
HCO_3: 23.2mmol/l
BE: −1.9

Billy was commenced on 40% oxygen via a face mask and monitored every 15 minutes on the ward. Later that afternoon his condition deteriorated further. On assessment ('Look: Listen: Feel: Measure'), he was:

increasingly breathless but his respirations were more shallow; centrally cyanosed; drowsy but rousable.

T: 38°C, R: 33/min, P: 110/min, BP: 95/60mmHg and SaO_2 : 78%

His oxygen flow was increased to 60%, but his ABG result confirmed he was experiencing life-threatening hypoxic respiratory failure:

pH: 7.33
PaO_2: 5.5kPa
$PaCO_2$: 4.7kPa
HCO_3: 20.4mmol/l
BE: −3.8

Billy was exhausted and drowsy, and met the criteria for mechanical invasive ventilation shown in Table 3.5. He was immediately transferred to ICU where he was intubated and supported with MIV.

Mechanical invasive ventilation in adults can only take place when a patient is intubated with a cuffed endotracheal or tracheostomy tube. The cuff provides a seal around the tube and prevents leaks. The purpose of MIV is to push air under pressure into the patient's lungs to ensure there is effective movement of oxygen and carbon dioxide in and out of the lungs (pulmonary ventilation). There are increasing numbers of types and modes of MIV, but for the purposes of this chapter we will limit discussion to two core modes: pressure-controlled ventilation and volume-controlled ventilation (Carbery, 2008; Grossbach et al., 2011). In Table 3.6 you will find an explanation of these modes together with the advantages and disadvantages of both.

In both pressure-controlled and volume-controlled ventilation the patient's respiratory rate can be managed in one of three ways.

*   The patient breathes spontaneously and controls their own rate.
*   The patient's respiratory rate is set and controlled by the machine.
*   The patient's respiratory rate is supported by a minimum respiratory rate set by the machine and supplemented by the patient's own respiratory rate.

The option of as much or as little respiratory support through MIV allows the patients to be as involved as possible in the process of respiratory support and aids their readiness to wean from MIV as they improve.

MIV mode	Risks	Benefits
Pressure-controlled / pressure-support ventilation: air is pushed into the lungs until a preset alveolar pressure is reached. For example: • Bilevel positive airways pressure (BiPAP) (see NIV). • Continuous positive airways pressure (CPAP) (see NIV). • Pressure-support ventilation (PS). • Positive end expiratory pressure (PEEP).	Ineffective ventilation. Hypo ventilation and variable tidal volumes triggered by reduced lung compliance in the presence of acute lung injury, sputum and/or bronchospasm. Compliance measures the 'ease of stretch' ability in the lungs. The more compliant the lungs are, the less pressure is required to open the airways during MIV.	Reduces the risk of ventilator-associated lung injury.
Volume-controlled ventilation: a preset volume of air is delivered to the lungs with each breath. For example: • synchronised intermittent mandatory ventilation (SIMV).	Ventilator-associated lung injury • Barotrauma: over-distension of some alveoli. • Volutrauma: over-distension of the alveoli caused by large tidal volumes. • Biotrauma: the release of inflammatory mediators that may increase patient mortality.	The machine delivers a set tidal volume with each breath, thus improving overall ventilation.
Modes that deliver a combination of both. For example: • pressure-regulated volume-controlled ventilation.		Reduces the risk of ventilator-associated lung injury. Ensures effective tidal volumes and pulmonary ventilation

Table 3.6: A comparison of pressure-controlled and volume-controlled ventilation modes

Case study: Billy Brown in ICU

When Billy arrived in ICU the intensivist and nurse explained to him that he was getting very tired and needed help with his breathing. They explained that he would need a tube inserted into his mouth so that air could be blown into his lungs. He wouldn't be able to speak with the tube in, and a nurse would be at his side 24 hours a day. He nodded. Billy had said on admission to hospital that there was no one he wanted to contact, no next of kin. Billy was sedated with intravenous propofol (a short-acting anaesthetic agent) and was given a muscle

continued . . .

relaxant to facilitate safe intubation with a low profile, cuffed oral endotracheal tube (size 8.5fg). He was attached to MIV using bilevel positive airways pressure ventilation (BiPAP). The parameters were:

Preset respiratory rate: 18/min
Preset inspired airway pressure: 30cm H_2O
Preset expired airways pressure: 15cm H_2O
Oxygen flow at 100%

The plan for Billy was to:

- *increase PaO_2 to >8.0 kPa;*
- *reduce the work of breathing so that he could rest;*
- *reduce the risk of alveolar collapse caused by inflammation and consolidation in the alveoli (see Table 3.3, pp55–6).*

ABGs sampled 30 minutes after the commencement of MIV illustrated that the first of these objectives had been achieved:

pH: 7.28
PaO_2: 22.9kPa
$PaCO_2$: 5.7kPa
HCO_3: 19.6mmol/l
BE: −6.9

Billy's oxygen flow was reduced to 80%. There is evidence to suggest that the use of 100% oxygen for more than six hours can damage lung tissue (Dunlop and Whyte, 2010). Billy's ABGs also showed that he had a metabolic acidosis caused by the presence of pancreatitis and sepsis.

Billy required MIV for a total of 24 days after having been diagnosed with acute respiratory distress syndrome (ARDS). Acute respiratory distress syndrome is a form of acute respiratory failure that leads to life-threatening hypoxia, inflammation, oedema and fibrosis in the alveoli. In Billy's case ARDS occured secondary to acute pancreatitis. On day 4, the oral endotracheal tube (ETT) was replaced by a tracheostomy. Initially, Billy was very distressed by the oral ETT and he required large doses of sedation and pain relief to help him cope. The intensivist estimated that this larger than normal amount was associated with Billy's high tolerance levels to alcohol and recreational drugs (de Wit et al., 2007).

Research summary: Sedation

The aim of using drugs to sedate patients during MIV is to promote comfort, relieve distress and anxiety, and facilitate effective respiratory function. The majority of drugs used for this purpose, however, can cause side effects, including: depression of the cardiovascular system leading to reduced BP; respiratory depression and delayed weaning from respiratory support; reduced motility of the gastro-intestinal tract with delayed absorption of nutrients; and poor quality sleep (Intensive Care Society, 2007; San Diego Patient Safety Council,

2009). The use of sedation assessment scales and sedation protocols have been recommended as a method for getting the balance right between the advantages and disadvantages of using sedation. The Ramsay scale, Riker Sedation-Agitation scale and Richmond Agitation and Sedation scale are examples of tools adapted for patients on MIV (Ramsay et al., 1974; Riker et al., 2001; Ely et al., 2003). There is limited evidence, however, that such scales and protocols can improve patient outcomes (O'Connor et al., 2010; Williams et al., 2008). There is evidence, however, that daily sedation interruption combined with patient assessment can improve patient outcome (O'Connor et al., 2008).

Gradually Billy's condition began to improve, and by day 16 he was awake and able to respond to commands, he was requiring less sedation and pain relief, and he was beginning to make the effort to breathe, although he still required help with MIV (BiPAP).

Preset respiratory rate: 14/min
Billy's own respiratory rate: 8/min
Preset inspired airway pressure: 28cm H_2O
Preset expired airways pressure: 8cm H_2O
Oxygen flow at 50%

Billy's ABGs on day 16 showed that he was no longer experiencing hypoxia or metabolic acidosis, although the damage to his lungs was manifested by a higher than normal level of carbon dioxide:

pH: 7.45
PaO_2: 11.4kPa
$PaCO_2$: 6.6kPa
HCO_3: 27.6mmol/l
BE: +3.4

Why are tidal volume, respiratory rate and airway pressure important in promoting optimum ventilation?

The tidal volume (TV) is the volume of air in each breath and can be measured as inspired (ITV) and expired (ETV) tidal volume. The respiratory rate (R) describes the total number of respirations in a minute. If a patient is on MIV this may include set ventilator breaths and the patient's own breaths. Minute volume is the total volume of air either inspired (IMV) or expired (EMV) in one minute and is equal to tidal volume times respiratory rate (Hall, 2011). Airway pressure is the same as alveolar pressure and is the pressure required or allowed to push air into the patient's lungs.

When assessing and monitoring a patient receiving MIV, tidal volume, rate, minute volume and airway pressure are some of the important indicators for measuring effective ventilation. For example, increasing ITV, R or IMV can improve the elimination of CO_2. If, however, by doing this the inspired airway pressure goes above 30–35cm H_2O, then the patient becomes at risk of acute lung injury. Patients such as Billy often develop reduced lung compliance due to inflammation and fibrosis of the alveoli, and it becomes harder to push air into the lungs. Promoting effective patient ventilation therefore requires assessment, monitoring, communication and collaboration with the patient, nurse, intensivist (anaesthetist) and physiotherapist to promote optimum lung function, and with the dietitian to promote optimum nutrition to support the patient's metabolic requirements and promote recovery (Woodrow, 2012). A summary of the risk assessment and management of patients such as Billy is illustrated in Table 3.7.

Risk assessment	Nursing interventions

Airway
• Risk of the endotracheal tube/tracheostomy (tube) occluding due to poor humidification, the patient biting down on the tube and/or secretions.
• Risk of airway irritation.
• Risk of the tube becoming dislodged.
• Risk of unplanned extubation.
	• Look for evidence of distress and agitation such as coughing and biting on the tube, assess the patient's sedation score and reassure. If the patient continues to be distressed, there is a higher risk of unplanned extubation and/or trauma to the patient's airways. If necessary, increase the sedation according to the prescribed guideline until the patient is comfortable.
	• Humidification of the airways can be achieved by:
	  • heat/moisture exchange (HME) filters that are attached to the ventilator circuit close to the endotracheal tube;
	  • hot water humidifiers (37°C);
	  • cold water humidifiers.

Breathing • Risk of airways becoming partially occluded leading to a rise in airway pressure and ineffective ventilation. • Risk of air leak due to poor connections. • Risk of inappropriately set alarm parameters. • Risk of ventilator-associated lung injury and ventilator-associated pneumonia (VAP).	• Narrowing or occlusion of the patient's airway can be identified by an increase in the inspired airway pressure and evidence of patient agitation, rattling/bubbling on chest auscultation. • Endotracheal suction is used to remove secretions in the trachea but should only be performed when there is evidence of the above. Suction can be painful, distressing and increase the risk of infection and trauma to the airways. • A loose connection can be identified by a reduction in inspired airway pressure, tidal volume, and reduction in SaO_2. • Assess respirations, inspired and expired tidal volumes and airway pressure, SaO_2 and ABG analysis if the patient's condition changes. • Set alarm limits to between 5 and 10 marks above and below the prescribed range and assess the patient hourly. • Adhere to the ventilator bundle.
Circulation • Risk of impaired circulation and cardiac function: MIV increases venous return pressure because the right side of the heart has to pump	• Assess the patient's vital signs for evidence of impaired circulation using continuous monitoring: heart rate and rhythm; BP; CVP; chest X-ray; signs of venous thrombosis; urine output, which should be ≥ 0.5ml/kg/hr (> about 30ml/hr).

Table 3.7: Risk assessment and plan of care for a ventilated patient

Continued

Risk assessment	Nursing interventions
against a higher alveolar pressure, thus raising the patient's CVP. Left ventricular cardiac output is reduced due to more blood staying in the venous circulation. Thus the patient is at risk of hypotension and oedema. • Risk of liver dysfunction leading to clotting disorders, immuno-suppression and reduced albumin production.	• Adhere to the ventilator bundle to reduce the risk of VAP. • Assess the patient for signs of peripheral oedema, bruising. • Assess blood results including: serum electrolytes; urea and creatinine; liver function tests; clotting. • Assess and screen for sepsis daily (Chapter 7).
Disability. • Inability to communicate verbally due the endotracheal tube and sedation. • Risk of pain. • Risk of poor skin integrity, dry eyes and mouth. • Risk of anxiety, delirium and/or boredom.	• When appropriate, encourage the patient to use non-verbal means of communication, picture cards and alphabet cards. Use eye contact and explain all procedures before they are attempted. • Assess the patient's pain using non-verbal cues and pain scores and manage appropriately. • Assess the integrity of the patient's eyes and mouth hourly and manage appropriately according to each patient's needs. • Adopt the Institute for Health Care Improvement (IHI, 2009) care bundle for pressure ulcer prevention: risk assess on admission; reassess daily: inspect skin, manage moisture on the skin, optimise nutrition and hydration, minimise pressure through positioning. • Help the patient to be orientated to night and day, and assess for signs of delirium (Chapter 8). • Encourage family-centred care and patient-focused care (Chapter 11). • Encourage the patient to be involved in decisions and, where possible, life outside the unit.
Exposure and safe environment. • Risk of infection associated with the use of invasive procedures. • Risk of noise and the environment disturbing sleep and rest.	• Risk assess and manage the patient with due regard to the ventilator bundle and risk assessment for sepsis. • Assess noise levels and reduce noise pollution where possible. Reorientate the patient to their environment and offer reassurance when appropriate.

Table 3.7: Continued

Concept summary: care bundles

Evidence-based practice is concerned with ensuring that the best available evidence is applied to practice. One method for achieving this is through the use of care bundles. Care bundles are a group of evidence-based interventions that, when combined, provide the most clinically effective method for reducing risk and improving patient outcome (Fulbrook and Mooney, 2003). The ventilator care bundle is an example of how combining selective interventions appears to have reduced the incidence of ventilator-acquired pneumonia (Lawrence and Fullbrook, 2011). The bundle combines the following four elements.

- Elevation of the head of the bed to 30–45%.
- Periodic interruption of the patient's sedation and daily assessment of the patient's readiness for extubation.
- Peptic ulcer disease prophylaxis.
- Venous thromboembolism prophylaxis.

Overall, Billy Brown was in ICU for 30 days. On day 24 he was awake and orientated, he was no longer on any sedation and his respiratory support had been reduced to the following.

Preset respiratory rate: 0
Billy's own respiratory rate: 21/min
Preset inspired airway pressure: 10cm H_2O
Preset expired airways pressure: 5cm H_2O
Oxygen flow at 40%

Look: Listen: Feel: Measure
Alert and orientated
Able to cough and expectorate sputum
No evidence of breathlessness or dyspnoea
T: 37°C, R: 21/min, P: 89/min, BP: 115/60mmHg and SaO_2: 97%

ABGs sampled were within the normal range
pH: 7.45
PaO_2: 13.2kPa
$PaCO_2$: 5.2kPa
HCO_3: 25.8mmol/l
BE: +2.5

Billy was waiting to have his tracheostomy removed and breathe on his own unaided for the first time in nearly a month. With Billy's cooperation the tracheostomy tube was removed and a secure dressing applied over the site. After six days Billy was well enough to be transferred to the ward, and a week later he was found accommodation in a hostel where he continued his rehabilitation.

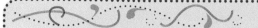

Chapter summary

In this chapter you have been introduced to patients who need advanced respiratory support. The technology and assessment strategies for patients in these situations are often complex, and the patient's condition can change suddenly. The important messages to gain from this chapter are as follows.

- Always begin by assessing the patient's airway, breathing and circulation, disability and environment, and you will always be able to prioritise care and communicate your concerns.
- Interpretation of the patient's condition through blood gas analysis means much more if the results are assessed in the context of the patient's story.

Activities: brief outline answers

Activity 3.1: Decision-making (pages 52–3)

Using the step-by-step guide in Table 3.2, what can you interpret from the arterial blood gas result?

These are the first set of ABG results.

- Joseph was showing signs of hypoxaemia on 60% oxygen.
- pH 7.07: shows evidence of acidosis.
- $PaCO_2$: 14.1kPa shows evidence of respiratory acidosis.
- HCO_3: 20.5mmol/l shows evidence of metabolic acidosis also.

Joseph's deterioration appeared to be due to a combination of respiratory acidosis caused by type II respiratory failure and a metabolic acidosis probably associated with his cardiac arrest.

What are your priorities of care for this patient?

- Joseph needs to receive support for his respiratory failure and should be assessed to determine the most suitable treatment plan. This may be a combination of nebulised short-acting beta agonist, short-acting muscarinic antagonist and intravenous antibiotics. He should be encouraged to sit up in the most comfortable breathing position and be assessed for NIV.
- Your role is to risk assesses the patient and reassure him, and if he is commenced on NIV, to support him to promote his comfort.
- If he is to be commenced on NIV, you will need to determine whether this will take place on the medical ward or whether he will be transferred to ICU and this will involve assessing Joseph's severity of illness and a skill mix assessment.

Joseph was reviewed four hours later. Using the step-by-step guide in Table 3.2, what can you interpret from the arterial blood gas result?

Joseph had been transferred to ICU for NIV following his assessment above and was commenced on bilevel positive airways pressure.

- Joseph's oxygen levels had improved and he continued on 60% oxygen.
- His pH of 7.30 is still showing signs of acidaemia.
- $PaCO_2$: 6.70kPa still shows evidence of respiratory acidosis but is much improved from his previous results.
- HCO_3: 25.7mmol/l shows evidence of a resolved metabolic acidosis.

Joseph's ABG's still indicate evidence of type II respiratory failure, but in this case his condition is improving.

What are your priorities of care for this patient?

- Joseph will require continuous assessment of his respiratory function with a view to reducing the NIV support over the next few hours if his condition continues to improve.
- He will need continued support and reassurance to maximise the effect of the respiratory support.

Further reading

Moore, T and Woodrow, P (2007) *High dependency nursing care: observation, intervention and support for level 2 patients*, second edition. London: Routledge.

This book offers practical help with learning how to use the technology when involved in the care of level 2 patients.

San Diego Patient Safety Council (2009) *Tool Kit: ICU sedation guidelines of care*. San Diego: San Diego Patient Safety Council. Accessed at: www.chpso.org/meds/sedation.pdf

This document gives you a helpful introduction to some of the drugs used to promote safety and pain relief for patients with mechanical ventilation. It also gives you examples of some of the assessment tools available for monitoring pain and sedation.

Useful websites

www.ics.ac.uk/intensive_care_professional/standards-safety_and_quality

The Intensive Care Society site provides access to relevant innovations and standards that relate to the care of patients who are critically ill. The website is multidisciplinary and offers information to patients and relatives in user-friendly guides.

www.ihi.org/offerings/initiatives/Pages/default.aspx

The Institute for Health Care Improvement website *Improvement Map* offers evidence-based and practical ways in which to provide safe and effective care for patients with acute and critical care needs.

Chapter 4
The patient with chest pain

David Barton with Thomas Barton

NMC Standards for Pre-registration Nursing Education

This chapter will address the following competencies:

Domain 3: Nursing practice and decision-making

3.1. Adult nurses must safely use a range of diagnostic skills, employing appropriate technology, to assess the needs of service users.

4.1. Adult nurses must safely use invasive and non-invasive procedures, medical devices, and current technological and pharmacological interventions, where relevant, in medical and surgical nursing practice, providing information and taking account of individual needs and preferences.

7.1. Adult nurses must recognise the early signs of illness in people of all ages. They must make accurate assessments and start appropriate and timely management of those who are acutely ill, at risk of clinical deterioration, or require emergency care.

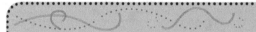

NMC Essential Skills Clusters

This chapter will address the following ESCs:

Cluster: Medicines management

34. People can trust the newly registered graduate nurse to work within legal and ethical frameworks that underpin safe and effective medicines management.

35. People can trust the newly registered graduate nurse to work as part of a team to offer holistic care and a range of treatment options of which medicines may form a part.

Chapter aims

By the end of this chapter, you should be able to:

- identify common causes of chest pain;
- distinguish symptom complexes in different kinds of chest pain;
- critically examine vital signs and understand other related investigations;
- identify and prioritise the most appropriate clinical nursing interventions;
- identify patient concerns and needs wider than those of the presenting chest pain.

Introduction

As a nurse, you will frequently work with patients who present with chest pain. Despite being a common presentation, it is also one of the most alarming for the patient and their family because most people associate chest pain with having a heart attack. The heart is the most vital of organs: we can feel it beating and hear its activity, and we all know that if it stops, this will quickly lead to death. However, a nurse must understand a great deal more about the causes of chest pain, as these can be many, commonly of cardiovascular, musculoskeletal, gastric or respiratory origin. A key intention of this chapter is to provide some insights on the more common causes of chest pain, how they may be identified and how they may be appropriately managed (ICSI, 2009). This chapter also explores the crucial part that the nurse, and teams of nurses, play in prioritising and managing interventions and care that enable recovery.

We will look at four patient scenarios that are typical of chest pain presentations. While the scenarios are condition based, you can follow the logical prioritisation of nursing interventions that are vital in managing such presentations. This will include those interventions required from the onset of the patient's chest pain through to those interventions that will enable a full recovery. In order to do this you will need to develop and apply your knowledge of nursing assessment, your ability to identify clinical signs, and your ability to formulate a reasonable nursing diagnosis based on symptom complexes and on underlying pathophysiology. No less than this will be your professional responsibilities of care, your identification of patients' physiological, psychological and wider social needs, and the demand for collaborative working when planning and implementing interventions and care.

As you work through each scenario you will note that we have not necessarily given comprehensive information on every aspect of the patient's needs, or all the information that may have been gleaned by the nursing assessments. We hope that you will pick up on these omissions, as there are activities where you will be able reflect on this. It will be you (the nurse) who should be seeking out and identifying these 'wider' concerns that extend beyond the patient's immediate presenting symptoms. Each of the scenarios is divided into three sections.

- The case history.
- The assessment of the presenting condition.
- Immediate and ongoing management of the presenting condition.

Possible causes of chest pain

The most common causes of chest pain are:

- cardiovascular disease (ischaemic coronary artery disease, conduction and rhythm disorders, congenital disorder);
- respiratory disease (chronic obstructive pulmonary disease, asthma, cancer, pneumothorax);
- musculoskeletal disorder or injury (mechanical injury, trauma);
- gastro-intestinal disease (gastritis, infection, herniation, pancreatitis and gall bladder disease);
- psychological causation (emotional disturbance, mental health disorder).

How do you assess and prioritise care for patients with chest pain?

Assessment of the patient experiencing chest pain, and the crucial information that arises from this, is vital in enabling the nurse to prioritise nursing interventions. It is undertaken using the normal tools and criteria that are used in any patient assessment: an initial primary assessment, followed by a comprehensive patient health history, including medications and symptom presentation, all coupled with baseline vital signs. It is important to remember that information may be gained from several sources: from the patient and their family; and from other members of the care team such as doctors, nurses, health care assistants and physiotherapists. What is crucial is that all this information is properly collated and acted on in an appropriate way by all members of that multidisciplinary team (MDT).

This assessment – shown in the box 'Taking the patient history' – will enable the nurse to prioritise the most immediate interventions to assure the patients well-being. In an acute presentation of chest pain, significant interventions will almost always include ongoing monitoring of vital signs – see the box 'Vital signs' – undertaking electrocardiographs (ECGs), administering prescribed medication, and ensuring a high standard of information and communication with the patient and all members of the MDT.

Taking the patient history

The primary nursing assessment is always 'Look: Listen: Feel: Measure'.

Taking a full patient history is a structured and systematic process. You should follow a format to ensure you gain as full a picture of the patient as possible.

- The presenting complaint (What is the problem? What are the presenting symptoms as reported by the patient and/or family?).
- The history of the presenting complaint (When did it happen? Where did it happen? How did it feel? What happened then?).
- Medications (current or old).
- Social history (a general review of the patient's social situation, family, employment, housing, etc.).
- Past medical history (a review of the patient's previous medical history).
- A family history (a review of the patient's family medical history).
- A general systems review – nervous system, musculoskeletal, heart, lungs, bowels, renal (Do you have headaches, any aches and pains, any chest or heart problems? How is your appetite? How are your bowels? Are you passing urine?).

Vital signs

The primary nursing assessment is always 'Look: Listen: Feel: Measure'.

Recording vital signs is a fundamental aspect of clinical data collection, and is a core component of the overall assessment. The core vital signs that are most commonly recorded are:

- respiratory rate;
- pulse;
- blood pressure;
- temperature;
- oxygen saturation;
- significant results – bloods, X-ray, scans.

Taking vital signs is *not* a one-off activity, and the regime of further measurements will depend on the patient's condition and the expert judgement of the medical and senior nursing staff.

Respiratory causes of chest pain

Case study: Mr Adams

Mr Adams, a 57-year-old man who has retired early, has attended his local GP's surgery as he has become increasingly short of breath during a summer heat wave. His wife insisted that he saw his GP. He tells the receptionist that he is feeling very unwell, that he has chest tightness and a generalised dull pain in his chest. He is asked to wait and told that a doctor will see him very soon. Shortly afterwards, following a spasmodic episode of coughing, he collapses in the waiting room. The receptionist reports to the attending practice nurse that Mr Adams became suddenly very short of breath and was wheezing, and that he had attempted to use an inhaler prior to collapsing on his chair.

The practice nurse makes an immediate initial visual and verbal assessment of Mr Adams, and finds him to be conscious but clearly in distress. He appears flushed and sweaty, is breathing noticeably quickly and has an audible wheeze. He can speak in short sentences only, but with assistance he can be helped to a wheelchair and moved to another room to be assessed. This immediate assessment informs appropriate interventions and the urgency of the presenting condition.

In a quiet room, Mr Adams manages to take his inhaler himself and appears to settle slightly. The practice nurse records his clinical observations – these affording an important baseline – and they are as follows.

- *Respiratory rate: 28bpm (audible wheezing).*
- *Pulse: 100bpm (regular, bounding).*
- *Blood pressure: 140/78.*
- *Temperature: 37°C.*

Activity 4.1   *Critical thinking*

- Are these observations normal? What do you make of these observations?

An outline answer to this activity is given at the end of the chapter.

The practice nurse undertakes a more detailed assessment of Mr Adams's recent health history – this is important in developing a more detailed picture of the patient. Mr Adams reports that he has chronic bronchitis, having previously been a heavy smoker, and that he has been short of breath and coughing more than normal for a couple of days. He feels the hot weather is making his shortness of breath worse and has had to use his inhalers more frequently the past couple of days. He is also treated for hypertension and high cholesterol, and he is overweight. In recent years his chronic bronchitis has become more severe and led to long periods off work before he retired. He is well known to the GP. Due to the sudden collapse of Mr Adams, and his distressed state, the practice nurse makes the decision that an immediate priority is that he requires constant observation. She stays with him, monitoring his respiratory status and offering him reassurance.

One of the surgery's GPs arrives and takes a full medical history, and performs an examination of Mr Adams. This reveals that, in addition to the practice nurse's observations, Mr Adams has also been coughing up some green sputum for the past two days.

The details of the GP's examination of Mr Adams are that:

- he is breathless at rest;
- he is using his accessory muscles to breathe;
- he has poor chest expansion;
- he is peripherally warm;
- he is cyanosed (appears blue).
- when auscultated, he has quiet breath sounds with a wheeze throughout his lung fields. He also has some basal crackles.

Activity 4.2   *Critical thinking*

- Given this information, at this point what do you think is causing Mr Adams's chest pain?

An outline answer to this activity is given at the end of the chapter.

Management of the presenting condition

The GP diagnoses Mr Adams with infective exacerbation of his chronic bronchitis. The immediate action necessary is urgent admission to hospital. Because of his collapse and the severity of his presentation, the GP wants Mr Adams to be admitted to hospital as a priority for initial investigation and treatment of acute exacerbation of chronic bronchitis.

Following admission to hospital, a first nursing priority is to ensure that he remains closely monitored given that he has collapsed as a result of his respiratory difficulties. The other clinical findings (green sputum) suggest he may have an infection, and his history suggests it is getting worse – he requires further and immediate investigations (Bridges and Dukes, 2005). The hospital nurses will need to ensure that the interventions listed below are quickly organised and undertaken so that appropriate therapeutic interventions can be commenced as soon as possible. The further investigations needed are:

- chest X-ray;
- sputum sample;
- blood tests – FBC, U&E and CRP.

These investigations will indicate the location of his infection (chest X-ray), the type of infection (sputum) and the severity of the infection (bloods). They may also highlight any other developing problems or otherwise undiagnosed issues. A next priority for nursing care is to initiate and provide the treatments prescribed, to monitor their effects, and to oversee the patient's care pathway.

Treatments and care planning

- Antibiotics, broad spectrum as per local health provider policy, which should be reviewed when a positive sputum culture is available.
- Bronchodilators, which will improve the patient's symptom of shortness of breath and hopefully reduce care requirements by allowing independence.
- Corticosteroids, which may be useful in COPD patients whose symptoms are not controlled by bronchodilators but should be stopped if there is no significant clinical improvement.
- Oxygen if clinically required – and only in small concentrations as higher concentrations can disrupt the patient's reverse drive respiratory effort and worsen their condition. If they remain unwell or are deteriorating with low concentration oxygen, then specialist respiratory medicine opinion should be sought.
- Discharge when improving.

Activity 4.3   *Communication and team working*

- While Mr Adams was awaiting admission from the GP surgery to hospital, what other wider concerns should the practice nurse be considering?

An outline answer to this activity is given at the end of the chapter.

Musculoskeletal causes of chest pain

Case study: Mr Knight

Mr Knight, an 82-year-old widower and a frail gentleman, has been admitted to a Clinical Decision Unit (CDU) for 24 hours' observation and monitoring of chest pain, having fallen at home tripping over his cat. He has fallen on to the left side of his chest and has had excruciating pain since. He was referred to hospital by his GP following a home visit; the GP was subsequently concerned when he noted that Mr Knight was on warfarin.

In CDU the nurses admit and undertake a primary assessment, quickly followed by a full nursing assessment including a systematic patient history and baseline vital signs. That assessment reveals that Mr Knight takes warfarin, digoxin, simvastatin and calcium tablets. Mr Knight tells the nurses that he is worried he is having a heart attack as a result of the fright, and he is clearly very anxious. In addition, it is noted that Mr Knight is lying on a bed wincing with pain and guarding the left side of his chest. It is painful for him to move, and he feels better when he is lying still. He is an articulate man, talking in full sentences, and he does not appear to be having problems breathing. He says he has awful pain in the left of his chest; it is constant and sharp,

continued . . . •••

throbbing in nature and made worse on deep inspiration. The nurses noted baseline vital signs. His observations are as follows.

- *Respiratory rate: 18bpm.*
- *Pulse: 90bpm (irregular).*
- *Blood pressure: 120/54.*
- *Temperature: 36.7°C.*
- *Oxygen saturation: 98.*

Activity 4.4   *Critical thinking*

- Are these observations normal? At this point, what do you make of these observations?

An outline answer to this activity is given at the end of the chapter.

Mr Knight tells the nurses that he knows he has had an irregular heartbeat for some time and this is why he takes warfarin (as his GP tells him he could have a stroke).

An on-call junior doctor takes a full medical history and examines Mr Knight. It is ascertained that he has fallen quite accidentally and has not felt dizzy, faint, blacked out, had palpitations or otherwise lost consciousness before or during his fall. He has pain that is isolated to the left side of his chest – it does not radiate anywhere and he does not feel short of breath. He does find it painful to take deep breaths. The medical examination finds that:

- he is a thin, frail man;
- he is pale;
- he has very extensive bruising and some swelling to the left side of his chest;
- the left side of his chest is painful when palpated;
- there is reduced chest expansion on the left.

Activity 4.5   *Critical thinking*

- With the information gained from the initial nursing assessment and with this information from the medical assessment, what do you now think is causing his chest pain?

An outline answer to this activity is given at the end of the chapter.

Management of the presenting condition

The doctor diagnoses Mr Knight with a haematoma and suspects possible rib fractures.
The immediate action taken is to:

- give analgesia;
- cannulate.

Now that Mr Knight has been assessed, it is a priority for the nurses to administer suitably strong prescribed analgesia for his pain before he goes on to have further necessary investigations (listed below). The nurses fully assess his pain both before and after administration of analgesia using a pain scale, but also with particular regard for any effect on respiratory effort. In addition, with evidence of bleeding and anaemia, it would be prudent to gain intravenous access early, and the nurses should ensure that cannulation is undertaken as soon as possible.

The further investigations undertaken are:

*   blood tests – FBC, U&E, INR, COAG;
*   chest X-ray;
*   12-lead ECG.

These investigations will identify with certainty if Mr Knight is anaemic as a result of his haematoma, or indeed by an as yet unidentified internal bleed (FBC). The COAG and INR tests will identify how thin his blood is and the clinicians may make a decision to actively reverse the effects of his warfarin. The blood tests may also identify evidence of underlying infection (often a precipitating factor of falls in the elderly). The chest X-ray will either confirm or exclude rib fractures, haemothorax or pneumothorax, and will likely show the haematoma in the soft tissues of his chest. The nurses will need to perform an ECG; this is prudent to rule out myocardial injury that may be masked by his musculoskeletal injury symptoms.

Treatments and care planning

*   Treatment will depend on the extent of bleeding. If anaemic, Mr Knight may require a transfusion of blood; if less anaemic than expected, a course of iron supplements may be prescribed.
*   Prompt administration (if required) of drugs such as beriplex and vitamin K will be required to reverse the effects of the warfarin (and help prevent further bleeding).
*   Rib fractures tend to be treated conservatively with analgesia and rest.

The CDU nursing will now need to ensure that Mr Knight is admitted to a ward bed as soon as possible where a full care pathway will be instigated. Key parts of that will include close monitoring of vital signs, pain management and appropriate mobilisation. A significant rationale for this is the potential for stroke, a major risk in elderly patients with AF (atrial fibrillation), and this will be exacerbated by the necessity of stopping warfarin in the light of his bleeding. It is crucial that the nurses note that his risk of stroke is very high, and that it is therefore important that he is closely monitored. Once his bleeding has stopped and he is stable, it is likely the clinicians will restart warfarin.

In addition, the ward nurses must note that with elderly patients who may develop a tendency to fall, the risk of intracranial bleeding with warfarin as a result of a head injury also becomes an issue. These situations are difficult and the patient should be fully investigated regarding the cause of their falls as current evidence suggests that all but the most prolifically falling patients should be maintained on warfarin as instance of stroke consistently outweighs that of intracranial haemorrhage.

Mr Knight presents a complex case for nursing management throughout, given his frailty, poly-pharmacy and multiple underlying health problems. Prioritising nursing interventions will be a pivotal part of Mr Knight's care pathway – with a central aim of enabling his eventual discharge. Full and ongoing nursing assessment, coupled with input from the MDT will ascertain the best time for discharge. Given his age and frailty, he may require temporary support at home, and the nurses will need to be sure that a package of care is ready for implementation on discharge home.

Activity 4.6 — Critical thinking

- Consider what other social and community issues the nurses may have had to think of.

An outline answer to this activity is given at the end of the chapter.

Gastric/abdominal causes of chest pain

Case study: Mrs Thompson

Mrs Thompson is an 81-year-old lady with dementia who lives in a nursing home. She complained of 'very bad' indigestion after her Sunday meal. Although forgetful and unable to live on her own as a result, Mrs Thompson is generally able to express herself well, and she told the nursing staff at the nursing home that she had severe pain in her chest. The nursing home staff called an ambulance to take her to A&E as they were concerned that she might be having a heart attack.

On admission, the A&E nurses assist Mrs Thompson to a trolley in the general waiting area of the emergency department. They carry out an immediate primary nursing assessment and note that she is clearly uncomfortable, sitting upright and burping a lot. She says she feels nauseous and that she has a very uncomfortable spasmodic burning-type chest pain. This pain is not radiating elsewhere. Her vital signs are as follows.

- *Respiratory rate: 22bpm.*
- *Pulse: 110bpm (regular).*
- *Blood pressure: 155/100.*
- *Temperature: 36.2°C.*
- *Oxygen saturation: 95%.*

Activity 4.7 — Critical thinking

- Are these observations normal?
- At this stage, what do you make of these observations?

An outline answer to this activity is given at the end of the chapter.

The A&E nurses note that Mrs Thompson is cooperative. She is able to mobilise with nursing assistance. A full nursing assessment (patient history and vital signs) is undertaken, coupled with an A&E doctor's physical examination and history. These reveal that:

- she is an elderly frail woman with mild cognition deficits;
- she is pale, but sweaty;

- she has a clear chest with normal heart sounds;
- the ECG reveals sinus tachycardia;
- her abdomen is tender on palpation, but no abnormal masses are identified;
- she has had mild diarrhoea for two days;
- she is on regular Gaviscon for persistent 'heartburn'.

Activity 4.8   *Critical thinking*

- With this information, what do you think is causing her chest pain?

An outline answer to this activity is given at the end of the chapter.

Management of the presenting condition

Mrs Thompson is experiencing an acute exacerbation of her chronic gastritis. The medical treatment of gastritis and the related prioritisation of nursing intervention will depend on what the underlying cause is (diet, infection, other medications such as asprin, **NSAIDs**, steroids). However, a first nursing priority for Mrs Thompson is to alleviate the symptoms; this is undertaken via administration of antacids and H-2 antagonists as prescribed. It is important that the nurses monitor and record the effects of these. Correction of electrolyte and hydration deficits will also be important, and a resultant nursing intervention will focus on administration of prescribed fluids and careful fluid balance monitoring.

Treatments and care planning

As Mrs Thompson is elderly and frail she will be admitted briefly for some investigations to explore possible underlying abnormalities that could be leading to her symptoms. The nursing teams will need to ensure that these investigations are planned and undertaken as soon as possible, and these will include:

- blood tests: blood cell count, presence of *H. pylori*, liver, kidney, gallbladder and pancreas functions;
- urinalysis;
- stool sample, to look for blood in the stool;
- chest and abdominal X-rays;
- repeat 12-lead ECGs.

Activity 4.9   *Reflection*

- Consider what other wider concerns the nurses should be thinking of in regard of Mrs Thompson's total care and return to her nursing home.

An outline answer to this activity is given at the end of the chapter.

Cardiac causes of chest pain

Case study: Harry Smith

*Harry Smith is a 58-year-old retired manager, married and a grandfather. He was diagnosed with type 2 diabetes when he was 48 years old. Harry began smoking when he was 15 years and only gave up smoking 40 cigarettes a day when he was diagnosed with diabetes. He had given up completely by the age of 50. Harry also suffers from hypertension and **hyperlipidaemia** and has been prescribed an ACE inhibiter (**angiotensin converting enzyme** inhibiter) to reduce his blood pressure, statins to reduce his blood cholesterol and aspirin to reduce the risk of clot formation. Harry is known to be at high risk of developing acute cardiovascular disease (NICE, 2008).*

Harry generally doesn't enjoy physical exercise, but he does enjoy gardening, and on the morning of his admission he had decided to start the first grass cut of the spring. Halfway through the job he developed central chest pain and he rested until the pain subsided. Not willing to leave a job half done, Harry went back outside to finish the grass. Later that afternoon Harry's wife came home to find him collapsed in the chair with severe central crushing chest pain.

Following an urgent admission via ambulance to A&E, Harry was immediately seen by A&E nurses and doctors and diagnosed with a primary myocardial infarction due to occlusion of a coronary artery. The ECG revealed evidence of ST elevation in the chest leads from V2 to V5, and Harry's troponin levels were elevated above the accepted reference limit.

The A&E nurses quickly assessed Harry's condition on admission. They found the following.

- *Respirations: 22/min.*
- *Pulse: 110, sinus tachycardia.*
- *BP: 110/80.*
- *Temperature: 37.5°C.*
- *SaO_2: 96%.*
- *He was pale and anxious.*
- *He had central chest pain and a 'heavy' left arm.*

Activity 4.10   *Critical thinking*

- Are these observations normal?
- What do you make of these observations?

An outline answer to this activity is given at the end of the chapter.

Management of the presenting condition

Harry was compensating for the loss of cardiac output by increasing his heart rate and respirations. A major nursing priority was to relieve his pain, which subsequently would alleviate ongoing stress on the heart. Pain assessment using a pain scale is a nursing priority. Harry was prescribed diamorphine to relieve the chest pain; this was administered by the nurses with measurable good effect. He was also prescribed aspirin to prevent further platelet aggregation and oxygen therapy to support an SaO_2 between 96 and 98%. He was booked for immediate angiography and percutaneous coronary intervention (PCI) within 90 minutes of admission to A&E (ICSI, 2009).

Monitoring fluid balance is a crucial nursing intervention in the patient with compromised cardiac function, and it was noted that Harry had not yet passed urine. The nurses inserted a urinary catheter, which drained 90ml of urine. He had last passed urine while at home before the onset of his symptoms.

Remember

Always 'Look: Listen: Feel: Measure'.

Ongoing management of the presenting condition

Just prior to transfer for angiography the A&E nurses reassessed Harry and found the following.

- BP 83/55.
- SaO_2 85%.
- His skin was cold and clammy.
- He was confused.
- He had central cyanosis.
- He was nauseated.

Activity 4.11   *Critical thinking*

- Are these observations normal?
- What do you make of these observations?

An outline answer to this activity is given at the end of the chapter.

Harry was presenting with the clinical features of uncompensated and progressive **cardiogenic shock**. Cardiogenic shock or cardiac shock is a clinical state where the cardiac output (volume of blood ejected from the left ventricle) is reduced, leading to inadequate perfusion of blood to the tissues, triggering the shock response. This can also be described as pump failure.

The most common cause of cardiogenic shock is myocardial infarction, when 40% of the heart muscle in the left ventricle has been damaged and the patient experiences failure of the left ventricle (Gowda et al., 2008). Other causes include severe contusion or bruising to the myocardium or a ventricular septal defect that reduces the efficiency of the left ventricular chamber as a pump. Cardiogenic shock can also occur in patients who develop septic shock and this is discussed in Chapter 7.

Regardless of the cause, the onset of cardiogenic shock triggers a cycle of events that lead to a continuing decline in cardiac function. Patients who develop cardiogenic shock often present with dramatic and distinctive features including:

- pale and cyanosed;
- confused and disorientated;
- feeling cold and clammy to touch;
- increased respiratory rate, tachycardia and hypotension.

Treatments and care planning

It is a priority that the nurses caring for Harry continue with a full systematic regime of ongoing regular assessment from the outset. The rationale for this is that patients such as Harry may be admitted to A&E with clinical features already present, but in many cases the cardiogenic shock may develop between five to seven hours after the onset of chest pain and the initial myocardial infarction (Babaev et al., 2005).

Harry's presentation and past medical history highlight a number of factors that increase the risk of patients developing cardiogenic shock.

- He has a history of diabetes.
- He has had a large anterior-lateral myocardial infarction, including ST elevation across his chest leads (V2–V5).
- He has an elevated troponin level.

The extent of ST elevation suggests that the damaged area involves both the front (anterior) and side (lateral) sections of his left ventricular myocardium and could involve 40% of his left ventricle.

Harry should remain in the resuscitation unit of A&E until they are ready to receive him in the cardiac catheter suite and/or operating department. He will need to be closely monitored every 15–30 minutes for a change in his condition. Following PCI or additional cardiac surgery Harry will require support in the Coronary Care or Cardiac Intensive Care Unit. Here nurses will provide continuous highly specialist support.

Further treatments and care planning

For Harry, the large area of ischaemia and inflammation to his heart muscle (myocardium) in the left ventricle caused by the coronary occlusion has led to reduced blood pressure and cardiac output. This has happened because the reduction in blood flow and oxygen available to the heart has led to a reduction in the energy available to support cardiac contraction. As a consequence Harry has reduced perfusion of vital organs and tissues.

The physiological response to shock in Harry's case would involve the triggering of the flight/fight response, including nervous and hormonal responses. This includes stimulation of the sympathetic nervous system to increase heart rate and peripheral vasoconstriction and the release of epinephrine (adrenaline) and norepinephrine (noradrenaline). However, due to the damage to Harry's heart, his body is unable to compensate for the reduction in cardiac output, and in spite of an increase in heart and respiratory rate, his blood pressure is below the level required to achieve adequate tissue perfusion. With no intervention the progressive reduction in blood pressure will continue, leading to the progressive stages of shock, including a further reduction in cardiac output, metabolic acidosis, further myocardial depression, loss of consciousness and reduced urine output.

The initial clinical priorities of care for patients in Harry's situation are the same as for acute coronary syndrome and that is to restore tissue perfusion in order to stabilise and facilitate recovery of the damaged myocardium. For Harry, restoring the circulation to the muscle damaged by the coronary occlusion will prevent the continual cycle of deterioration into cardiogenic shock.

Heart muscle will begin to die through the process of necrosis and form scar tissue if the blood supply is not restored within four to five hours after injury. The primary treatment for patients in cardiogenic shock, therefore, is PCI and restoration of blood flow. This has been demonstrated to improve the long-term survival rates of patients such as Harry when compared to medical stabilisation alone (Hockman et al., 2006).

In order to stabilise Harry for safe transfer to the operating department medical stabilisation is first required. The nursing priorities for this will include:

- providing oxygen therapy to restore SaO2 to 98%;
- instituting and monitoring of prescribed fluid resuscitation to improve vascular circulation;
- administration and monitoring of intravenous drugs to improve cardiac function (**inotropic therapy**) such as **dobutamine**, **dopamine** and milrinone (see Chapter 7).

If Harry's condition does not respond to PCI or if he is unsuitable for reperfusion therapy with thrombolytic drugs (dissolving the blood clot) or coronary artery bypass surgery, medical support will be the most effective option (Babaev et al., 2005). In this case Harry may need the support of non-invasive ventilation (NIV) and intra-aortic counterpulsation. The nursing management of such complex procedures will be undertaken within high-dependency areas.

The provision of intra-aortic counterpulsation involves the insertion of a catheter into the aorta. The catheter has a balloon at the distal end and during cardiac diastole (ventricular relaxation) the balloon will inflate. This creates a back pressure during ventricular relaxation that will improve the blood supply to the coronary arteries that branch off the aorta above the catheter tip. During cardiac systole the balloon deflates and creates a reduction in peripheral resistance, thus reducing the workload of the left ventricle and improving cardiac output.

Harry was commenced on oxygen therapy and received fluid resuscitation. An intravenous anti-emetic was prescribed and administered by the nurses to relieve the nausea. He was transferred immediately to the cardiac catheter suite and underwent PCI with the insertion of two stents to the left anterior descending artery. A stent is a 'stainless' tube that, when inserted and guided into place with a cardiac catheter, expands and pushes against the inner (endothelial) layer of the coronary artery, expanding the diameter of the artery and improving blood flow to the ischaemic myocardium.

The key interventions responsible for Harry's recovery were:

- timely assessment and diagnosis;
- fast and efficient communication;
- the work of the paramedical staff that transferred him to A&E;
- efficient and thorough nursing and medical assessment in A&E, and early recognition and reporting of his deterioration to the cardiology team;
- cardiology intervention;
- critical care support – specialist nursing care.

Activity 4.12   *Reflection*

- With appropriate intervention, Harry will be able to return home. What do you think the main issues that the nurses should consider in enabling the 'journey' to recovery when Harry goes home?

An outline answer to this activity is given at the end of the chapter.

Following the PCI Harry's condition began to improve. His blood pressure quickly improved to 90/60 and he became less confused and cyanosed. Over several days his condition continued to improve and he was discharged from hospital eight days after the onset of his chest pain. Prior to discharge Harry was commenced on a rehabilitation programme that focused on reviewing and improving diet, exercise and medication to reduce the risk of further cardiac problems.

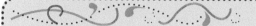

Chapter summary

This chapter has presented four clinical scenarios that have highlighted different causation of chest pain. The first three demonstrate how chest pain may arise as a result of other factors than myocardial infarction. This is not comprehensive, and we have not delved into other less common reasons such as adverse drug side effects or anxiety related issues. The final scenario, however, has presented a classical, and serious, presentation of chest pain that is directly related to cardiac disease.

Key points that must arise from this are:

- the need for rapid and full systematic nursing assessment;
- the need for prioritisation of initial nursing interventions;
- the need for nurses to take immediate and regular ongoing vital signs;
- the need to keep an open mind on the cause of 'chest pain';
- the need for holistic nursing assessment throughout the patient journey.

We hope that you take from this chapter, if nothing else, the knowledge that there may be many causes of 'chest pain, and many means of assessing and intervention.

Activities: brief outline answers

Activity 4.1: Critical thinking (page 75)

The respiratory rate is very high for a man of this age at rest; the pulse is slightly elevated; the blood pressure is within a normal range for a man of this age; the temperature is on the border of elevation above normal.

Activity 4.2: Critical thinking (page 76)

This symptom complex is highly suggestive of a chest infection that is exacerbating ongoing lung disease.

Activity 4.3: Communication and team working (page 77)

Mr Adams's wife will need to be contacted and given information regarding his prospective admission, and an opportunity to ask questions or attend the surgery to be with her husband. The nurse should be responsive to her expected concern and anxiety. In addition the nurse should be able to provide information as to where Mr Adams will be first admitted – most likely to a medical admissions unit.

Activity 4.4: Critical thinking (page 78)

The respiratory rate is slightly evaluated; his pulse would not be considered abnormal in a man of his age – later investigation revealed underlying atrial fibrillation treated with digoxin and warfarin; blood pressure is slightly low for a man of his age; temperature is within a normal range; oxygen saturation is normal.

Activity 4.5: Critical thinking (page 78)

With a history of a fall, this information is highly suggestive of trauma – a potential haematoma – and could point to rib fractures. The nurse should be aware of the potential for pneumothorax and monitor respiratory function closely.

Activity 4.6: Critical thinking (page 80)

You should have picked up on two key issues – the first leading you to the second. First, Mr. Knight tripped over his cat: who would be available to care for the cat while he was in hospital? Second, the scenario does not provide any information on his social status. Does he live alone? Does he have family? How accessible is his accommodation for the shops? Does he have friendly neighbours? What is his financial situation? Does his accommodation need modification to make it safer for him? Will there be a requirement for community nursing or community health care support? Your reflection on Mr Knight should have taken in these wider holistic concerns.

Activity 4.7: Critical thinking (page 80)

The respiratory rate is elevated; the pulse is elevated – tachycardia; the blood pressure is moderately high – particularly the diastolic; the temperature is normal; the oxygen saturation is acceptable for the patient's age.

It would be difficult in isolation to make any conclusion from these readings. However, in conjunction with other findings they would evidence a patient experiencing pain.

Activity 4.8: Critical thinking (page 81)

These findings are highly suggestive of acute or chronic gastritis – and further enquiry would reveal that Mrs Thompson has a history of persistent heartburn.

Activity 4.9: Reflection (page 81)

A significant issue for this woman is her dementia. The scenario presents her as very cooperative – but as increasingly forgetful. There is also a real possibility that dementia may worsen in future. An important issue that arises from for nurses planning discharge to the nursing home will be ensuring that the nursing home understands her problems. Dietary advice will need to be given to minimise episodes of gastritis, this coupled with a carefully monitored regime of H-2 antagonists and antacids.

Activity 4.10: Critical thinking (page 82)

The respiratory rate is significantly high; the pulse is elevated – tachycardia at rest; the blood pressure is low, even for a known and treated hypertensive; the temperature is above the normal range; the SaO_2 is acceptable.

Central chest pain radiating to the left arm accompanied with pallor is typically suggestive of myocardial infarction, although this could only be confirmed in the light of other investigations.

The observations point to a physiological state of compensating shock.

Activity 4.11: Critical thinking (page 83)

The blood pressure is significantly low from the previous baseline; the SaO_2 is significantly low; this clinical profile points to a developing physiological sate of decompensating shock.

Activity 4.12: Reflection (page 85)

Harry was commenced on a rehabilitation programme while still an inpatient and will continue that programme following discharge home. The key elements to cardiac rehabilitation programmes focus on improving diet, exercise and appropriate medication management. Support and compliance with all of these will help to reduce the risk of further cardiac problems.

Chapter 5
The patient in pain

Catherine Williams with Susan Salerno

NMC Standards for Pre-registration Nursing Education

This chapter will address the following competencies:

Domain 3: Nursing practice and decision-making

Generic competencies:

3. All nurses must carry out comprehensive, systematic nursing assessments that take account of relevant physical, social, cultural, psychological, spiritual, genetic and environmental factors, in partnership with service users and others through interaction, observation and measurement.

6. All nurses must practise safely by being aware of the correct use, limitations and hazards of common interventions, including nursing activities, treatments, and the use of medical devices and equipment. The nurse must be able to evaluate their use, report any concerns promptly through appropriate channels and modify care where necessary to maintain safety. They must contribute to the collection of local and national data and formulation of policy on risks, hazards and adverse outcomes.

Field-specific competencies:

3.1. Adult nurses must safely use a range of diagnostic skills, employing appropriate technology, to assess the needs of service users.

NMC Essential Skills Clusters

This chapter will address the following ESCs:

Cluster: Organisational aspects of care

9. People can trust the newly registered graduate nurse to treat them as partners and work with them to make a holistic and systematic assessment of their needs; to develop a personalised plan that is based on mutual understanding and respect for their individual situation, promoting health and well-being, minimising risk of harm and promoting their safety at all times.

10. People can trust the newly registered graduate nurse to deliver nursing interventions and evaluate their effectiveness against the agreed assessment and care plan.

continued . . .

Cluster: Medicines management

36. People can trust the newly registered graduate nurse to ensure safe and effective practice in medicines management through comprehensive knowledge of medicines, their actions, risks and benefits.

38. People can trust the newly registered graduate nurse to administer medicines safely and in a timely manner, including controlled drugs.

Chapter aims

By the end of this chapter, you should be able to:

*   discuss the anatomy and physiology of pain transmission;
*   define acute and chronic pain;
*   effectively assess pain using a variety of assessment tools;
*   reflect on clinical examples in the chapter and apply this to your own clinical situation.

Introduction

This chapter is about the physical and psychological impact of pain, and will explain how you perform an accurate pain assessment. It will explain the importance of monitoring patients using clinical assessment skills and procedures.

Pain is sometimes considered to be the fifth vital sign after temperature, pulse, respiration and blood pressure (Lynch, 2001) and should form an integral component of your nursing assessment. Pain can have harmful physiological, psychological and emotional effects on your patient. Many patients in the clinical environment experience pain, which is usually related to surgery, trauma or some form of organ disease.

Case study: Jackie's story

*Maddie, a student nurse, is on a placement in the Burns Unit and is working with her mentor on admissions. One evening a patient called Jackie is transferred for assessment to the Burns Unit. She has sustained a 12% scald to both legs while draining a pan of pasta. She is still in a great deal of discomfort despite receiving a total dose of 30mg of intravenous morphine (in increments of 10mg) and paracetamol 1g intravenously prior to transfer from A&E. The medical staff are reluctant to give further opiates at present as they are concerned that this will cause respiratory depression. However, Jackie is asked to assess her pain level on a scale of 0–10 and rates the pain as 11. Maddie's mentor explains that the patient's nerve endings have been left exposed to the air by her injury and that the uncovering of the wound for assessment is contributing to Jackie's discomfort. The mentor also explains that the wound will have to be cleaned and debrided prior to dressings being applied and that this is likely to make the pain worse, albeit temporarily. The mentor then becomes an advocate for the patient and suggests to the medical staff that she might benefit from using **nitrous oxide** for pain relief until the wound can be covered. Checks are made with the patient and there are no contraindications for her to receive this form of analgesia. The mentor sets about explaining to Jackie how to use the nitrous oxide*

continued . . .

inhalation system. Jackie has used nitrous oxide in childbirth, and the wound assessment and dressings are able to proceed. When the wounds are properly dressed and no longer exposed to the air, Jackie's discomfort abates and she is able to breathe normally and no longer requires the nitrous oxide.

The aetiology of pain

Wilson (2007) describes acute pain as being a physiological response that warns us of a threat or danger to the body. Because of the increase in hormone production and sympathetic output in the body from injury or illness, your patient, when in pain, will experience an increase in heart rate and blood pressure, which increases cardiac work and oxygen consumption.

This physiological response comes from the nervous system that directs and manages the functions of all the cells and tissues in our body. In short, the theory is that a stimulus activates the nerve ending pain receptors, and this stimulus is known as a **nociceptor**.

For example, if you burn your finger, the tissue damage activates the nociceptors, which in turn transmit impulses to the brain via the spinal cord causing you to experience **nociceptive pain**.

Another type of pain stimulus is known as **somatic pain**, which is a type of nociceptive pain. The nerves that detect somatic pain are located in the skin and deep tissues, and they send impulses to the brain when they detect some kind of tissue damage, for example, if you cut your finger, stretch a muscle too far or exercise for a long period of time. The pain experienced will be sharp due to the tissues being rich in the A delta (A) fibres sending rapid signals to the brain, and this is why you are able to clearly locate the origin of the pain and it usually causes you to cry or scream.

Pain from deeper tissues is known as **visceral pain**. Visceral pain is also a type of nociceptive pain, but it originates from the internal organs. Like somatic pain, the nociceptors send signals to the spinal cord and brain when damage is detected. Visceral pain is often described as generalised aching or squeezing in the body. For example, if you suffer from irritable bowel syndrome or bladder disorders, you will experience visceral pain. The generalised aching or squeezing felt is caused by compression or stretching of the abdominal cavity. Visceral pain can radiate to other areas in the body, which is why pinpointing its exact location can be difficult.

Activity 5.1	*Critical thinking*

Research nociceptive, visceral and somatic pain in more depth. Try to identify the specific areas of the body that may be affected, what type of injury may cause them in a patient and how the pain for each area may be experienced.

There is no outline answer provided for this activity.

Types of pain

When treating patients you always need to consider the type of pain that they are suffering in order that you use the appropriate strategy to alleviate it.

Pain is classified as acute or chronic (Dougherty and Lister, 2008). **Acute pain** is normally of sudden onset, usually occurring as a result of tissue damage, injury or disease, and it tends to resolve over time as tissues heal. **Chronic pain** begins with an episode of acute pain, but unlike acute pain, chronic pain does not resolve over time. The most common causes of chronic pain are degenerative conditions such as osteoarthritis or diabetic complications such as neuropathy. Table 5.1 shows some common examples of chronic and acute pain.

Chronic pain	Acute pain
Diabetic neuropathy	Migraine/headache
Back pain	Burns
Osteoarthritis/rheumatoid arthritis	Fractures
Multiple sclerosis	Lacerations
Cancer	Abdominal pain
Neuralgia	Toothache
Post-surgical pain	Post-surgical pain

Table 5.1: Examples of chronic and acute pain

You need to be aware that some patients can suffer from both forms of pain (chronic and acute), and a number of nursing interventions that you routinely perform on your patient such as suctioning, line insertion, repositioning and physiotherapy can cause additional pain and discomfort.

Providing comfort to your patient who is in pain is a vital role of the nurse, and implementing supportive measures will minimise the overall pain and anxiety in your patient. Communication, reassurance, touch and explanations are important skills that you need to incorporate into your practice. Simple measures such as reducing noise levels and light, and relieving prolonged pressure or limb placement and turning pillows over may help relieve positioning discomfort in your patient and decrease anxiety levels.

Activity 5.2   *Decision-making*

Think about the scenario above. What type of pain do you think Jackie is suffering from? What is your reasoning for deciding this? What simple interventions could you introduce to help alleviate her anxiety and promote comfort?

An outline answer can be found at the end of the chapter.

Pain assessment

Assessment of pain is an important aspect of your role that requires a number of skills, including observation, interpretation and communication skills. Other interventions that can be used to assess pain include:

- analgesic administration;
- emotional support;
- cognitive techniques;
- comfort measures.

Pain assessment in patients is often poor because pain is an individual experience, but remember that the patient's response to pain can be affected by a multitude of variables such as age or culture, not just the type of pain and its duration.

Activity 5.3   *Reflection*

Think back to a time when you managed the care of patients who suffered moderate to severe pain. How did they express pain? Did they express their pain in the same way as other patients? If not, what were the differences?

There is no outline answer at the end of the chapter as this activity is based on your own reflections.

What should be covered in your pain assessment?

Your initial assessment of the patient's pain assessment should include:

- the underlying condition;
- whether the pain is acute or chronic;
- whether any medical treatment is being given;
- related symptoms such as vomiting and breathlessness;
- meaning or significance of the pain for the patient.

You can undertake an initial or ongoing assessment using a pain assessment tool. Many assessment tools are available, although the most commonly used pain scale in the health care setting is the numerical rating scale. The numerical scale offers the individual in pain an opportunity to rate their pain score. The user rates their scale from 0 to 10 when asked, or places a mark on a line indicating their level of pain. The lowest figure indicates the absence of pain, and the highest figure represents the most intense pain possible.

An advantage of the numerical scale assessment is that it follows the World Health Organisation (WHO) analgesic ladder (WHO, 1996). The WHO ladder provides a simple step-by-step guide to increase or decrease analgesics and its advantages include:

- simplicity – in that only a few, widely known drugs are employed;
- applicability – to a wide variety of situations and prescribers worldwide;
- safety – in that the safer drug is used first.

Activity 5.4   *Reflection*

Investigate the pain relief analgesic ladder devised by the WHO. Reflect back on a patient you have cared for who benefited from having their medication linked to the principles of the ladder.

There is no outline answer at the end of the chapter as this activity is based on your own reflections.

Another pain assessment method that is easy to remember is the PQRST mnemonic – which stands for Provokes, Quality, Radiates, Severity and Time (Skaer, 1998) shown in the box 'Pain recognition and assessment'. This method has five simple characteristics to help you in the questioning of the patient's pain assessment, but remember that you must let the patient describe the pain, as sometimes they say what they think you would like to hear.

Pain recognition and assessment

P = Provokes
- What causes pain?
- What makes it better?
- What makes it worse?

Q = Quality
- What does it feel like? Can you describe the pain? Is it:
- Sharp?
- Dull?
- Stabbing?
- Burning?
- Crushing?

R = Radiates
- Where does the pain radiate?
- Is it in one place?
- Does it move around?
- Did it start elsewhere and is now localised to one spot?

S = Severity
- How severe is the pain on a scale of 1–10? This can be a difficult one as the rating will differ from patient to patient.

T = Time
- Time pain started?
- How long did it last?
- Is it constant or does it come and go?

There are other assessments of pain you can use for patients who cannot use verbal or visual ratings scales (for example, if your patient is intubated). The Behavioural Pain Scale (BPS) is very useful in the assessment of pain in critically ill patients as it works by evaluating facial expressions, upper limb movements and compliance with mechanical ventilation.

Although not the ideal assessment, when used alongside other non-verbal signs such as blood pressure, heart rate and vasoconstriction, it can help indicate pain in your patient.

It is vital that you regard the patient's pain as an assessment priority. Unless pain is assessed regularly and effectively, your patient will continue to suffer unnecessarily.

Assessment in the very young, the cognitively impaired (such as the sedated patient or those with dementia) and those with communication problems can pose problems, but there are suitable pain assessment tools such as verbal rating, visual analogue, body diagrams, question-naires and pain diaries. The following are examples of validated pain assessment scales that are provided for your use via **www.npc.nhs.uk/therapeutics/pain**.

Effective pain assessment is a fundamental part of your nursing care, and the accountability of pain assessment lies firmly within the domain of nursing. To enable you to do this effectively, keep in mind the following.

- Seek to establish a relationship with your patient.
- Use open questions.
- Observe your patient for clues regarding pain.
- Avoid jumping to conclusions.

Activity 5.5   *Critical thinking*

Consider our case study patient Jackie. Of the assessments scales that have been discussed, which one do you think would be most appropriate for her, and why? What other factors will you observe in your assessment?

An outline answer to this activity is at the end of the chapter.

Managing your patient's pain

The choice of drug used to alleviate your patient's pain depends upon the nature and severity of the pain, and many other factors that the doctor will consider.

The three main classes of drugs that are commonly used within the hospital care environment are:

- non-opioids;
- opioids;
- anti-emetics.

We will now go on to look at each of these classes of drugs in more detail.

Non-opioids

This class of analgesics is better suited to treating musculoskeletal pain or mild to moderate pain generally associated with inflammation. Non-opioids are widely used and include aspirin, paracetamol, ibuprofen and diclofenac. Paracetamol is included in this group but has very weak anti-inflammatory effects. The route of administration will depend on your patient's condition. Take care to bear in mind your patient's renal clearance as **nephrotoxic** medication such as NSAIDs increase the risk of kidney failure. Non-opioid analgesics such as paracetamol and aspirin are readily available over the counter, though many stronger forms may require a doctor's prescription.

For further information and guidance on pharmacology and therapeutics of this group of drugs, you should refer to the *British National Formulary* (*BNF*: http://bnf.org/).

Opioids

Some prescription medicines contain drugs that are controlled under the Misuse of Drugs legislation. These medicines are called controlled drugs. Examples include: benzodiazepine, morphine, pethidine and methadone. Opioids originate from the opium poppy and are generally suitable for treating moderate to severe pain. They work by interfering with the transmission of the pain signal to the brain and change the way the brain perceives pain. However, potentially lethal side effects such as respiratory depression and changes in consciousness level mean that they must be appropriately selected, prescribed, administered and monitored. Opioids can be short-acting or long-acting, depending on how they are manufactured. Morphine is recognised as one of the strongest of opioid therapy; it relieves dull, prolonged pain and is long-acting, making it a good choice of drug for bolus administration. (Bolus administration is when a relatively large dose of medication is administered into a vein in a short period, usually within 1–30 minutes.)

Diamorphine is synthesised from morphine and works by mimicking the action of naturally occurring pain-reducing chemicals called endorphins. Pethidine is a synthetic form of morphine and has muscle-relaxant properties, but due to its very short-acting properties it is very rarely used in the ICU setting and more frequently used within a ward setting. Fentanyl is a synthetic opioid that is more potent than morphine and is not appropriate for general pain management due to its strength. Because it does not cause histamine release in your patients there is less risk of hypotension. Fentanyl derivatives include remifentanyl and alfentanyl.

Ketamine is a co-analgesic, and so is most effective when used alongside a low-dose opioid. It has analgesic effects in itself, although high doses can cause disorienting side effects, and it tends to increase heart rate and blood pressure.

Opioids can be administered via multiple routes but have many side effects such as respiratory depression, cough suppression, constipation, urinary retention, and nausea and vomiting, with the additional potential to depress the gag reflex, causing aspiration; hence, close observation and documentation is vital to prevent complications occurring.

For further information and guidance on the pharmacology and therapeutics of the above, please refer to the *British National Formulary* (*BNF*: http://bnf.org/).

Anti-emetics

You can buy some anti-emetics that help relieve nausea and vomiting over the counter without a doctor's prescription, but generally anti-emetics are prescription-only drugs

Many different types of drugs are used to control nausea and vomiting. Some affect brain function by preventing the stimulation of the vomiting centre, and others work on the gut by speeding up motility. The most commonly used anti-emetics such as ondansetron, prochlorperazine and cyclizine affect the vomiting centre, whereas metoclopramide increases gut motility. The patient's symptoms will affect the choice of anti-emetic.

For further information and guidance on the pharmacology and therapeutics of the above, please refer to the *British National Formulary* (*BNF*: http://bnf.org/).

Research the main analgesics listed above, using the *British National Formulary* (*BNF*) at http://bnf.org/ and ascertain the contraindications, interactions and side effects of these drugs.

Identify whether each of the drugs listed above are mild, moderate or severe analgesics in line with the WHO (1996) pain ladder.

There is no outline answer at the end of the chapter as this activity is based on your own research.

Activity 5.7   *Reflection*

Think about the burns patient, Jackie. How effective are these drugs likely to be for her? Why is the analgesia not working effectively? Is this to do with the type of injury, the choice of drug, or the individual?

An outline answer is given at the end of the chapter.

Epidurals

An epidural anaesthetic works by blocking the nerve roots that lead to the uterus and lower part of the body. The nerve roots are located in a space near the spinal cord called the epidural space. The epidural space extends from the base of the skull to the sacrum and the space is identified by feeling for bony landmarks on the spine and pelvis. A fine-bore catheter is inserted into the epidural space and the ligaments and bones of the spinal cord; the catheter is secured to the patient's back and then attached to the infusion device.

The area of analgesic effect is dependent on the site of insertion in relation to the surgery. Epidural location sites are:

- T6–T9 abdominal surgery – exploratory laparotomy;
- T7–T10 upper abdominal surgery – repair of abdominal aortic aneurysm;
- T9–L1 lower abdominal surgery – repair of inguinal hernias;
- L1–L4 hip and knee surgery.

(Dougherty and Lister, 2008)

The drugs most commonly used for epidural analgesia are opioids such as fentanyl and bupivacaine. Bupivacaine can be used on its own (usually for a bolus dose) and dosage will depend on the size of the catheter and the type of surgery. Remember that epidural analgesia is contraindicated in patients who have:

- local or systemic infection;
- known neurological disease;
- coagulation disorders or who are undergoing anticoagulant therapy;
- spinal arthritis/spinal deformities;
- hypotension;
- marked hypertension.

(Hastings, 2009)

What is epidural analgesia? Where is it administered? Discuss the specific nursing care associated with administering drugs via this route.

An outline answer can be found at the end of the chapter.

You always need to observe the epidural site for any signs of infection, inflammation and **phlebitis** during your assessment. When removing the epidural line, ensure you use a strict aseptic technique to reduce the risk of infection and haematoma. As a matter of good practice you should always check clotting time (PT 10–14 seconds) before removal and always check the catheter tip is intact after removal. Because of the risk of bleeding, avoid prophylactic heparin administration before and after removal of the line (times will be identified in your local policy); many clinical areas have specific step-down analgesia protocols that are implemented to avoid premature discontinuation – see your local policy for further guidance. Epidural use is usually limited to a maximum of four days because of the significant risk of infection after this period of time. Any concern you may have about the epidural site or infusion should be discussed immediately with the pain team or the anaesthetist.

As with all controlled drugs you must prepare, administer and document the drugs according to your hospital policy. For further information and guidance with regard to pharmacology and therapeutics of the above, please refer to the *British National Formulary* (*BNF*: http://bnf.org/).

Patient-controlled analgesia

Patient-controlled analgesia (PCA) is widely used for the treatment of pain in the ICU environment. The PCA offers on-demand, intermittent, IV administration of opioids under patient control (with or without a continuous background infusion). This technique is based on the use of a sophisticated microprocessor-controlled infusion pump that delivers a pre-programmed dose of opioid when the patient pushes a demand button; lock-out controls are set to prevent excessive administration or overdose.

Research PCA – what is it? What are the main advantages and disadvantages of its use in patients experiencing pain in hospital or the community?

There is no answer to this activity at the end of the chapter. The issues are discussed below.

Using a PCA system allows your patient more immediate relief of incidental (breakthrough) pain and can provide a greater sense of personal control over pain. It can be reassuring to your patient to know that an analgesic is quickly available and that they are in control of the administration.

As the opioid analgesia is not administered unless the patient presses the control, it is important that they are able to operate it properly. The PCA system will be unsuitable for a patient who does not have the cognitive ability to understand how to use the PCA device, or who is unable or unwilling to operate the hand set.

Because a strong opioid is being administered, you will need to have a clear understanding of the contraindications and therapeutics of the drug being administered and its side effects. As with epidurals, hourly checks of the following must be completed and documented:

- heart rate;
- blood pressure;
- respiratory rate;
- oxygen saturations;
- pain score;
- sedation score;
- nausea/vomiting;
- dose used.

In addition to your patient checks, pump checks need to be completed to enable continuing assessment. Pump checks include:

- programme check;
- amount delivered;
- successful attempts;
- unsuccessful attempts – *this will indicate that analgesic needs are not being met and the regime needs to be urgently reviewed*;
- lock-out time – the lock-out interval is designed to prevent overdose. Ideally, it should be long enough for the patient to experience the maximal effect of one dose before another is permitted.

A PCA is usually needed for a few days after surgery/medical interventions, and many ICUs have specific step-down analgesia protocols to prevent premature discontinuation and ensure patients remain pain free during the step down from intravenous to oral medication. Any concern you may have about the PCA infusion should be discussed immediately with the pain team or the anaesthetist.

As with all controlled drugs you must prepare, administer and document the drugs according to your local policy. For further information and guidance with regard to pharmacology and therapeutics of the above, please refer to the British National Formulary (*BNF*: http://bnf.org/).

Recognising deterioration in your patient

When you have a critically ill patient who has difficulty communicating their pain due to altered levels of consciousness (LOC) or endotracheal intubation, they may have a continuous infusion to prevent exacerbation of pain. Unfortunately, there are risks of over-dosage, especially in patients with kidney or liver dysfunction. You must report any changes in your patient's pain or overall condition. You will need to make frequent observations and assessments so that you spot any change in their condition or adverse effects caused by treatment. Be aware of patients receiving strong opiates and sedation for post-operative pain as they could be at risk of respiratory depression. You will need to assess pain and sedation hourly. When caring for a patient in pain, it useful to remember the following.

- Think of pain as the fifth vital sign – any increase in your patient's pain may mean deterioration in your patient's condition.

- Always report any new sources for pain identified by your patient – this could be a sign of surgical and/or medical complications.
- Opioids have strong side effects. Your patient will require specific and close monitoring and you may need to administer other drugs to overcome the side effects.
- Never focus solely on the one aspect of your patient's pain – take into account all possible factors that may be affecting their pain management.

Non-pharmacological pain management

Non-pharmacological approaches may contribute to effective analgesia, are often well accepted by patients and are a useful adjunct in managing pain. The role of non-pharmacological approaches to pain management is evolving, and it is likely that some non-pharmacological and complementary therapies may have an important contribution to make to holistic patient care. The goals of non-pharmacological interventions are to:

- minimise fear and distress;
- make pain more tolerable;
- give the patient a sense of control over the situation and their behaviour;
- teach and enhance coping strategies.

Common non-pharmacological pain-control methods widely used in hospitals and in the community are distraction, music therapy, hypnosis, cold and heat application, transcutaneous electrical nerve stimulators (TENS) and massage therapy. You need to be familiar with each of these methods. It is also important that you develop a therapeutic nurse–patient relationship and pay attention to comfort measures, as these will aid pain control in your patient. Fear and anxiety make pain worse, so your nursing care should aim to alleviate these feelings.

Scenario

Jackie is now at home recovering from her burns. You are on clinical experience with the district nurse who is visiting Jackie. What kinds of non-pharmacological interventions could you discuss with Jackie to manage her pain?

Non-pharmacological interventions that can be implemented to manage Jackie's pain are as follows: distraction, music therapy, hypnosis, transcutaneous electrical nerve stimulators (TENS) and cognitive behavioural therapy (CBT). Noise levels, lighting, and physical and psychological comfort should also be considered.

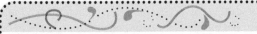

Chapter summary

Pain can be triggered by many medical conditions, including ischaemia, infections, inflammation, oedema, distension, immobilisation, incisions and wounds. The use of invasive and non-invasive medical devices can also cause pain in your patient. In addition, many commonly performed nursing procedures such as suctioning, turning, dressing *continued ...*

changes, and the insertion and removal of catheters may be a source of pain for your patient, and these need to be taken into consideration when assessing pain.

Preventing pain will improve your patient's physiological and psychological outcomes, enabling earlier discharge. Remember that pain is individual to each patient (McCaffery and Pasero, 1999) and will always require regular individual assessment. Pain is usually a symptom of a problem, and even though analgesia will be provided, the cause of your patient's pain will still need to be investigated. Unless pain is assessed regularly and effectively, the patient will continue to suffer unnecessarily.

Pain management has to be one of your top nursing priorities and you must continue to monitor outcomes related to pain management. Some patients may be able to verbally or non-verbally communicate their pain-control needs; the critically ill intubated patient may not be able to communicate their level of pain adequately, and this needs to be recognised in the care plan. To fulfil the above you will need to have a thorough understanding of the actions of analgesics, their side effects, dosages, and differing methods of administration and appropriate use within the ICU setting to ensure a positive outcome for your patient.

Activities: brief outline answers

Activity 5.2: Decision-making (page 91)

Jackie is suffering from acute pain. Burn pain is one of the most difficult forms of acute pain to treat. The type of tissue damage with a burn injury is likely to generate unusually high levels of pain.

Activity 5.5: Critical thinking (page 94)

Assessment tools are essential to the diagnosis of underlying burn pain syndromes and the effectiveness of their treatment. The better tool to use with this patient is one of the verbal self-report instruments that measure pain intensity, such as the '0–10' numeric rating scale. This is the most appropriate tool as assessing pain in the burn-injured patient is complex and as she is able to communicate well, this assessment tool will give you a clear picture of her pain status.

Activity 5.7: Reflection (page 96)

Burn pain is difficult to control because of its unique characteristics, its multiple components and its changing patterns over time. Cleansing wounds, changing dressings and providing physical therapy involve repeated manipulations of painful sites. Understanding the mechanisms that contribute to the intensity and variability of burn injury pain over time is crucial to its proper management.

Activity 5.8: Critical thinking (page 97)

An epidural is a form of regional analgesia involving an infusion of drugs through a catheter placed into the epidural space. Epidural analgesia may be administered either as a continuous infusion, as patient-controlled epidural analgesia (PCEA), or as a combination of the two. The injection can cause both a loss of sensation and a loss of pain by blocking the transmission of signals through nerves in or near the spinal cord. A comprehensive assessment should include vital signs, pain and sedation levels, level of consciousness, ability to void, sensation and motor function, presence of potential adverse side effects and complications, and evaluation of insertion site.

Your patient will require vital signs monitoring throughout its use for signs of hypotension (due to **vasodilation** of the vessels) and respiratory depression (due to opioid analgesia). Most clinical areas advocate an hourly protocol check of:

- heart rate;
- blood pressure – hypertension should not be managed by tilting the patient head down as this will allow the drug to travel up to T4 and cause paralysis of the respiratory muscles;
- respiratory rate;
- oxygen saturations;
- pain score;
- dose delivered;
- sedation score;
- nausea/vomiting – if your patient is complaining of a headache and nausea/vomiting, this may be a sign of a dural puncture;
- level of sensory/motor block – the block should be high enough to provide effective analgesia but not to paralyse the respiratory muscles. If this occurs, you must stop the infusion immediately;
- the dressing.

Further reading

Caudill, M (2008) *Managing pain before it manages you*, 3rd edition. New York: Guilford Press.

This book continues to be the gold standard for the self-management of pain. It is informative and easy to read, focusing on what people can do on their own to manage persistent pain.

Herndon D N (2007) *Total burn care*, 3rd edition. London: W B Saunders.

This book will give you a comprehensive overview of the assessment and management of a patient with moderate and severe thermal burns.

Mann, E and Carr, E (2006) *Pain management: essential clinical skills for nurses* London: Blackwell Publishing.

Pain management is a practical guide to current best practice, providing students and newly qualified nurses with the knowledge and skills required to care for a person experiencing or at risk of experiencing pain.

Useful websites

http://bnf.org/

Compiled with the advice of clinical experts, this essential reference provides up-to-date guidance on prescribing, dispensing and administering medicines.

www.britishpainsociety.org

This is a useful website for current information on all matters relating to pain.

www.nice.org.uk/

This website allows you to access a series of national clinical guidelines to secure consistent, high-quality, evidence-based care for patients using the National Health Service.

www.npc.nhs.uk/therapeutics/pain/overview

This is an easy, user-friendly website that provides summaries of the best available evidence relating to prescribing issues, and it will help you to critically review the evidence base for interventions and discuss the implications for the care of patients and best practice.

Chapter 6
The patient in shock

Desiree Tait with Bethan James

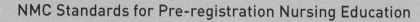

NMC Standards for Pre-registration Nursing Education

This chapter will address the following competencies:

Domain 3: Nursing practice and decision-making

3.1. Adult nurses must safely use a range of diagnostic skills, employing appropriate technology, to assess the needs of service users.

7.1. Adult nurses must recognise the early signs of illness in people of all ages. They must make accurate assessments and start appropriate and timely management of those who are acutely ill, at risk of clinical deterioration, or require emergency care.

Chapter aims

By the end of this chapter, you should be able to:

- identify the causes of shock;
- describe clinical features of shock and the clinical implications for the patient;
- differentiate between and diagnose possible causes of the patient's deterioration;
- demonstrate how to assess, record and respond to patients at risk of shock;
- demonstrate an awareness of risk assessment in the context of holistic care;
- reflect on clinical examples illustrated in the chapter and apply this to your own clinical situation.

Introduction

Case study: Jenny's story

Jenny, a third-year student nurse, was responsible for the management of six patients on a surgical ward under the supervision of her mentor. One of the patients in her care was Megan, a 75-year-old woman with a history of ischaemic heart disease and abdominal pain. She had been assessed by the surgical registrar, and the agreed plan was to withhold oral intake, commence intravenous fluids and monitor her progress. Jenny, after seeking advice from her mentor, commenced hourly observations of respiration, temperature, pulse and blood pressure. Several hours later she noticed Megan's blood pressure had gone down, with pulse and respiratory rate showing

continued . . .

a slight increase. All the changes occurred just within the normal range, however, and did not identify Megan as being at risk. Jenny contacted the house officer, who suggested that she should keep monitoring the patient and that they would review the patient on the medical round later that day. One hour later Megan collapsed, and she died that afternoon in the intensive therapy unit. The post-mortem revealed that Megan had died from shock induced by a perforated peptic ulcer.

Jenny's experience highlights that if a patient going into shock is not diagnosed and managed in a timely and effective manner, it can be fatal. Megan had been unwell for several days with abdominal pain, nausea and indigestion. She was dehydrated and had only drunk sips of water. Megan had been taking 75mg aspirin for ten years as part of her routine medication as well as anti-hypertensive drugs and statins to reduce her cholesterol. Jenny had been aware that one of the side effects of aspirin is bleeding in the gastro-intestinal tract but assumed that the house officer was aware of this. Jenny had identified that Megan's condition was changing and she had taken some correct steps to increase the monitoring of vital signs, but she had not taken into account all the signs that can indicate deterioration in a patient's condition. Jenny felt she had monitored her patient carefully, but she had failed to see the significance of the trend in Megan's vital signs and had not noticed or reported that Megan had become more restless and anxious. These signs were all indicative of a patient's deteriorating condition. The surgical team had assessed and reviewed the patient without knowing or attending to all the relevant clinical features. As a result, both nursing and medical staff failed to interpret, communicate and act on the available clinical evidence.

What can we learn from this?

Shock is a complex condition that can manifest in many different ways. The main aim in nursing care is to identify the symptoms of impending shock so that early indications can be interpreted and significant deterioration in a patient's condition prevented. There are important messages to learn from Jenny's story.

- Always be alert to changes in your patient's clinical condition, no matter how small.
- If you are concerned about a patient, always assess and record all the relevant details, including medical history, changes in the patient's appearance, behaviour and vital signs, and then communicate those concerns, guided by the SBAR communication tool (see Chapter 1, page 10).
- If you are still concerned, continue to seek advice and support according to local risk assessment protocol (see Chapter 1).
- Timing is of the essence: your patient will continue to deteriorate whether you wait or not.

This chapter provides an overview of the general causes and manifestations of shock and examines in detail the care of a patient with **hypovolaemic shock**. The underlying physiology, social psychology and ethical implications of the patient's care will be discussed in the context of risk assessment and collaborative management of care. The chapter proceeds with an overview of the knowledge and skills required to assess, differentiate and manage the care of patients who progress to clinical shock. The assessment and management of patients with cardiogenic shock are discussed in Chapter 4, and patients with distributive shock, including sepsis and **septic shock**, are discussed in detail in Chapter 7.

What is shock and why does it occur?

Shock is defined as 'a clinical state which occurs when an imbalance between oxygen supply and demand results in the development of tissue hypoxia' – a reduction in the supply of oxygen to the tissues (McLuckie, 2009, p97). For example, if a patient has a haemorrhage and loses 30% of their total blood volume, the patient will have insufficient levels of circulating blood to transport oxygen and nutrients to the body's cells. Without the oxygen and nutrients required for normal cell function, the body's organs and tissues will start to fail – this is known as tissue hypoxia (see Chapters 2 and 3). Initially, the patient's physiological systems will try to compensate by triggering the sympathetic nervous system and the flight/fight response.

We tend to see the flight/fight response as a biological response that is triggered in situations of perceived stress when the body will focus on providing energy and resources to the brain, heart and muscles to aid either running away from danger or standing and fighting. In the case of our haemorrhaging patient, the response is designed to keep the blood supply flowing to the tissues. If, however, the cause of blood loss in our haemorrhaging patient is not found and treated, the patient will continue to deteriorate and move to the progressive stage of shock, when the patient is no longer able to compensate for the amount of blood lost (the key stages are set out in Table 6.3 later in this chapter). At this stage the body is using all its reserves to try to maintain homeostasis, and if left untreated, the refractory stage of shock will be reached – the point when the body is no longer able to compensate for the blood loss and body organs start to malfunction due to tissue hypoxia. In Jenny's story, by the time Megan collapsed she was already in the progressive stage of shock, and in spite of last-minute support, she progressed to the refractory stage and died later that day in ITU.

You will come across shock in many clinical situations and different locations. A person may go into shock for a number of reasons – for example, physical trauma, dehydration, sepsis, anaphylaxis and haemorrhage. Such situations can occur in the person's home, outside, and in any hospital or care setting. In Megan's case shock was caused by loss of blood and body fluids, triggered by a perforated gastric ulcer, and is described as hypovolaemic shock. The types of shock are classified in four categories according to the underlying cause.

- **Hypovolaemic shock** due to decreased circulating blood volume.
- **Cardiogenic shock** due to impaired cardiac function.
- **Obstructive shock** caused by an obstruction to the circulating blood flow.
- **Distributive shock** caused by altered distribution of blood in the central and peripheral circulation.

(Mattson Porth and Matfin, 2009)

All of these situations will result in insufficient blood (and therefore oxygen and nutrients) to the cells. Table 6.1 lists the categories and common causes of shock in each category, with some clinical examples. Table 6.2 provides a summary of the clinical features that are present when patients are diagnosed with a particular type of shock.

Categories of shock	Causes of shock	Clinical examples
Hypovolaemic	Decreased blood/plasma/extra cellular fluid volume due to the following: 1. External haemorrhage. 2. Internal haemorrhage. 3. Trauma and fractures. 4. Severe vomiting and diarrhoea. 5. Dehydration. 6. Major burns. 7. Peritonitis/pancreatitis (inflammation in the peritoneal cavity or the pancreas).	1. Tom was stabbed in the leg and sustained an estimated blood loss of 750mls. 2. Terry Jones with haematemesis and melaena (see scenario on page 11) 3. Bill Holland sustained a fractured shaft of femur in a road traffic collision. 4. Mary has food poisoning. 5. Betty slipped and fell and has been lying on her kitchen floor for 2 days with no food or water. 6. Jane was trapped in her car as it caught fire and she sustained 80% burns. 7. Henry was admitted with acute abdominal pain, gallstones and pancreatitis.
Cardiogenic	Impaired cardiac function leading to reduced cardiac output and blood pressure due to the following: 1. Myocardial infarction (MI) (blocking of a coronary artery). 2. Myocardial contusion (bruising of the heart muscle). 3. Structural defects such as a ventricular septal defect (a hole in the wall of the septum between the right and left ventricles). 4. Cardiac arrhythmias (narrow and broad complex tachycardia).	1. Harry Smith is diagnosed with a large myocardial infarction and develops cardiogenic shock (see scenario on page 82). 2. Bill Holland sustained severe trauma to his sternum and myocardial contusion from the seat belt during the collision. 3. Fred recovered well from acute coronary syndrome until two weeks after treatment when he collapsed and was diagnosed with a ventricular septal defect secondary to a MI. 4. Jane was experiencing repeated episodes of broad complex tachycardia and her blood pressure had fallen to 80/35.

Table 6.1: Categories and common causes of shock

Continued

Categories of shock	Causes of shock	Clinical examples
Obstructive	Obstruction to the circulating blood flow due to the following. 1. Cardiac tamponade (bleeding or fluid between the myocardial and pericardial layers of the heart, causing the heart to be squashed). 2. Pulmonary embolus (obstruction of oxygenated blood back to the left side of the heart). 3. Tension pneumothorax (air leaking and trapped between the pleural layers of the lungs causing the lungs and heart to become squashed in the thoracic cavity.	1. Bert was one hour in to his post-operative care following cardiac surgery when he suddenly collapsed, becoming breathless and disorientated. 2. Janet had been complaining at home of a red and swollen leg for two days when she suddenly collapsed with chest pain and breathlessness. A deep vein thrombosis in her leg had travelled in the circulation to the lungs causing an obstruction in blood flow. 3. Sarah was a passenger on a flight from London to Florida when she suddenly experienced severe difficulty with breathing. The change in pressure during the flight had caused a tension pneumothorax in her right lung.
Distributive	Altered distribution of blood flow to the central and peripheral circulation. 1. Septic shock caused by Gram-positive bacteria/Gram-negative bacteria. 2. Systemic inflammatory response (SIRs) leading to vasodilation and body organ failure. 3. Anaphylaxis following exposure to an antigen. 4. Neurogenic caused by: a) cervical spinal cord injury leading to impaired function of the sympathetic nervous system and the flight/fight response; b) anaesthesia/sedation causing depression of the respiratory and circulatory system.	1. Angela had been admitted to the ward in a distressed and confused state, with severe hypotension and a diagnosis of severe sepsis secondary to a urinary tract infection. 2. Within an hour Angela's condition had deteriorated and she was admitted to ITU with septic shock and SIRs (see Chapter 7). 3. Helen was admitted to A&E in a collapsed state after being stung by a bee 20 minutes before. 4. a) Paul sustained injuries to his cervical spine and spinal cord as the result of his car overturning. His blood pressure was 80/40 and his pulse 50/min. b) Mary had been given a general anaesthetic for a surgical procedure, following which she had difficulty waking up, her respiratory rate was 10/min, pulse 55/min and BP 84/52.

Table 6.1: Continued

Assessment	Hypovolaemic	Cardiogenic	Obstructive	Distributive		Anaphylactic	Neurogenic
				Septic			
Look: Skin colour? Trauma/injury? Behaviour? Level of consciousness (LOC)?	Pale Tachypnoea Restless, anxious Blood or fluid loss Thirst	Grey skin with central and peripheral cyanosis Drowsy and confused Thirst	Grey skin with central and peripheral cyanosis Breathless Altered LOC Sudden onset	Initially flushed with vasodilation Pale and cyanosed later Exhaustion Confusion		Redness and swelling on face and neck Breathless/wheeze Blistering/Wheals/Pruritis Exposure to an allergen Fear/anxiety/Altered LOC	Pale Faint Altered LOC Post-anaesthesia/head/spinal injury
Listen: Patient/relative story? Past and recent history?							
Feel: Skin? Pulse?	Skin cool	Skin cold and clammy	Skin cool and clammy	Skin initially warm but then cold		Skin warm	Skin warm and dry

Table 6.2: A summary of the clinical features found on assessment of patients with different types of shock

If any of these signs are present the patient is at risk and should be risk assessed using track and trigger, sepsis screening and SBAR.

Continued

Assessment	Hypovolaemic	Cardiogenic	Obstructive	Distributive		Anaphylactic	Neurogenic
				Septic			
Measure:							
Respiration (R)	Tachypnoea	Tachypnoea	Tachypnoea	Tachypnoea		Tachypnoea	Bradypnoea
Pulse (P)	Tachycardia	Tachycardia	Tachycardia	Tachycardia		Tachycardia	Bradycardia
Blood pressure (BP)	Hypotension	Normal BP progressing to hypotension	Normal BP progressing to hypotension	Hypotension		Hypotension	Hypotension
Oxygen saturation (SaO$_2$)	Reduced SaO$_2$	Reduced SaO$_2$	Reduced SaO$_2$	Reduced SaO$_2$		Reduced SaO$_2$	Reduced SaO$_2$
Arterial blood gas analysis	Metabolic acidosis	Hypoxia	Hypoxia	Hypoxia as shock progresses		Hypoxia as shock progresses	Hypoxia as shock progresses
Pain score	Pain relative to cause	Pain relative to cause	Pain relative to cause	Metabolic acidosis			
LOC	Reduced CVP	Cardiac arrhythmias	Cardiac arrhythmias	Reduced CVP		Reduced CVP	Reduced urine output
ECG	Reduced urine output	Elevated CVP	CVP relative to cause	Reduced urine output		Reduced urine output	
Central venous pressure (CVP)		Reduced urine output	Reduced urine output	Fever with white cell count above or below the norm			
Urine output							

Table 6.2: Continued

If any of these signs are present the patient is at risk and should be risk assessed using track and trigger, sepsis screening and SBAR.

Activity 6.1	*Reflection*

With reference to Tables 6.1 and 6.2, think back to your experiences in the clinical setting and identify examples of situations where patients have been diagnosed as being in shock.

- Are any of the clinical situations you identified listed in Table 6.1?
- Did the patient deteriorate suddenly or over a period of several hours?
- What clinical signs and features were present to indicate your patient was in shock?

Hint: These reflective questions will help you to practise linking the causes and types of shock to the signs and symptoms present in the patients you have nursed.

There is no outline answer at the end of the chapter as this activity is based on your own reflections.

Shock, regardless of the cause, has a high incidence of morbidity and mortality that increases as the length of time before the patient is diagnosed and treated. Early recognition and anticipation of the potential for patients to develop shock is a key nursing activity that can lead to reduced morbidity and mortality of patients in your care (NICE, 2007a, 2010d; Tourangeau et al., 2006).

What are the stages and signs of shock?

In health, balance between the body's physiological systems is maintained through homeostasis. This process involves the purposeful control and maintenance of the body's organs so that normal body functions can continue efficiently. These integrated systems usually operate through negative feedback systems: physiological control mechanisms that respond to a change in the normal range of a substance by triggering other mechanisms until the uncontrolled substance is back within normal range (Hall, 2011). The effects can be manifested through physical, emotional and behavioural reactions to a stressor, such as haemorrhage. For example, using negative feedback, a fall in blood pressure will be identified by pressure sensors in the aorta and carotid arteries. A message will be sent to the brain via the autonomic nervous system that triggers the body to resist the fall in blood pressure by causing blood vessels in the peripheral circulation to constrict (patient becomes pale). As a consequence, the volume of blood in the central circulation will increase and ensure that the heart, brain and muscles receive oxygen. This can be described as the **initial stage of shock**, and in Megan's case this was demonstrated when Jenny noticed Megan's blood pressure had gone down, with pulse and respiratory rate showing a slight increase. All the changes occurred just within the normal range, however, and did not identify Megan as being at risk. At the time Megan had also become more restless and anxious, but the significance of this had been lost on Jenny and she was unable to connect the subtle changes in her patient's condition. Jenny's mentor, however, should have been able to interpret these changes and act on them by monitoring the patient every 10–15 minutes and seeking advice from the outreach team. This example highlights the importance of undertaking a holistic assessment and clinical interpretation of the patient's situation as well as having an awareness of the risks associated with the patient's illness.

Initially, the flight/fight response is able to support and compensate for impaired circulation and uptake of oxygen. Signs and symptoms of shock occur when the body's systems respond by increasing the pulse and respiratory rate, preserving body fluids by reducing urine output and attempting to maintain an effective supply of blood and oxygen to the tissues. This is known as the **compensatory stage of shock**. Support and management of the underlying cause can reverse the shock at this stage.

However, if the primary cause of the problem is not resolved or controlled, eventually the compensatory mechanisms will be unable to maintain effective circulation, and the patient will collapse, as in Jenny's story. This leads to ischaemia (decreased blood supply to the tissues) and tissue hypoxia (reduction in oxygen supply to the tissues). Without an adequate supply of oxygen, the cells will no longer be able to function effectively and will start to fail. This is known as the **progressive stage of shock**. When a patient enters the progressive stage of shock they are critically ill and need intensive support. It is during this stage that organ failure, such as acute renal failure and acute lung injury are likely to occur. Even with intensive support of the body's systems, the damage to body organs is likely to continue, leading to multiple organ failure. This is known as the **refractory stage** when shock becomes irreversible and the patient is likely to die.

Regardless of the type and cause of shock, if the patient does not receive the appropriate interventions, the ultimate outcome will be the same. However, with timely assessment and intervention, the effects of shock can be reversed before the patient progresses to the final and irreversible stage. The four progressive and interrelated stages of shock are presented in Table 6.3.

In the next sections we will consider the clinical features and signs at each stage in detail by following the care of a patient with hypovolaemic shock. In each section we will explore how you can assess and manage the patient in order to provide clinically effective care.

Hypovolaemic shock

Assessment and management of patients with hypovolaemic shock

As we have seen, hypovolaemic shock occurs as a result of the loss of a critical volume of blood, plasma or extracellular fluid. In a healthy adult male at a weight of 70kg the total blood volume is an estimated 4,900mls (70mls of blood/kg). This is the volume required to maintain an effective circulation (Mattson Porth and Matfin, 2009). If a patient loses up to 10% of their circulating volume, the body will respond and compensate so that no obvious clinical signs are evident. However, if the loss continues unabated, clinical signs will become evident when approximately 15% loss is reached. The greater the volume of loss, the more significant the clinical effects become and cardiac output decreases exponentially (Hall, 2010). When cardiac output falls, this means that there is a reduced volume of blood being pumped into the systemic circulation every minute. To try to increase the volume, the body will increase the heart rate. With continuing loss of blood or body fluids, however, the body finds the task of compensating for the loss more difficult. Table 6.4 illustrates the physiological impact of hypovolaemic shock caused by haemorrhage on the patient's clinical features, based on percentage of blood loss (American College of Surgeons, 2008).

External blood loss leading to hypovolaemia can be measured through visual estimation on examination of the patient and environment. For example, a patient with bleeding oesophageal varices (ruptured blood vessels in the oesophagus) will have a recent history of acute and severe haematemesis. When bleeding is internal, the pattern of evidence is more complex and can only be estimated on the basis of a physiological understanding of the patient's condition and

Stages of shock	Physiological and clinical progress	Patient example
1. Initial	• The body systems are able to accommodate the clinical trigger or cause. • Clinical features are often not apparent at this stage and the situation can go unrecognised. • Shock is reversible with assessment and intervention.	Mrs Brown has a two-day history of diarrhoea and vomiting. Her GP records her vital signs as: R: 18/min; P: 92/min; BP: 110/65. These are within the normal range; however, if her symptoms persist, she could go into hypovolaemic shock. He prescribes an intramuscular injection of anti-emetic to reduce the vomiting and suggests she contacts the surgery again tomorrow if she feels no better.
2. Compensatory	• If the cause remains active the body's physiological systems will be triggered. • Clinical features including an increase in pulse, respirations and a reduction in BP, and will be evident as the flight/fright response initiates a cascade of physiological responses in an attempt to compensate for the loss of homeostasis. • Shock is reversible with assessment and intervention,	The following day Mrs Brown's vital signs have deteriorated. The vomiting has subsided but the diarrhoea persists. She is anxious, cold to touch and thirsty. Her vital signs are: R: 20/min; P: 100/min; BP: 89/58.
3. Progressive	• The underlying cause and impact persists. • Physiologically the body has used all the compensatory mechanisms available in an attempt to return to homeostasis and has failed to compensate. • This leads to tissue ischaemia and hypoxia. • Shock is reversible in the early stages with appropriate assessment and management.	Mrs Brown was taken to the A&E unit where an assessment shows evidence of further deterioration. She is confused and agitated. She has not passed urine for 24 hours. Her vital signs are: R: 24/min; P: 110/min; BP: 80/50. Mrs Brown receives fluid resuscitation and management of the underlying cause. Her condition improves and within four days she is discharged home.
4. Refractory	• Physiologically the body has been unable to compensate, leading to cell death, tissue death and multiple organ dysfunction syndrome. • Shock is irreversible.	If Mrs Brown had not been referred to A&E in a timely manner by the GP, her condition would have continued to deteriorate and without support Mrs Brown would have become drowsy and eventually lost consciousness. She would have become peripherally and centrally cyanosed (see Chapters 2 and 3), and her vital signs would have been: R: 30/min; P: 120/min; BP: 65/40. She would be suffering from tissue hypoxia and renal failure.

Table 6.3: The stages of shock, illustrated by a clinical example

On assessment	Initial	Compensatory	Progressive	Refractory
Loss of blood or body fluid volume	0–15%, 750 ml	15–30%, 750–1,500 ml	30–40%, 1,500–2,000 ml	>40%, >2,000 ml
Look/ Feel	Minimal clinical signs	Cool skin	Pale, cool	Pale, cold to touch
Look/Listen	Anxious	Anxious	Confused and agitated	Loss of consciousness
Measure heart rate		Tachycardia	Tachycardia	Increasing tachycardia
Measure respiratory rate		Tachypnoea	Tachypnoea	Increasing tachypnoea
Measure blood pressure	Unchanged	Reduced BP and pulse pressure	Hypotension below systolic of 90mmHg	Severe hypotension, with narrow pulse pressure
Measure urine output			Oligurea	Oligurea progressing to anurea

Table 6.4: Stages of hypovolaemic shock based on percentage of blood/fluid loss for a 70kg male (for example, Terry Jones, case study, page 113)

following a clinical assessment and examination of the patient. For example, a patient with a fractured shaft of the femur can have an estimated blood and fluid loss of up to 2,000mls, while a patient with a traumatic fracture of the tibia can lose an estimated 800mls into the surrounding interstitial tissue around the site of the fracture. In this example both patients have a risk of developing shock, but the patient with a fractured shaft of femur will have a much higher risk of going into shock within 30 minutes of injury than the patient with a fractured tibia. This will be manifested by evidence of patient anxiety, pale cool skin, tachycardia, tachypnoea, and reduced blood pressure (difference measured between the systolic and diastolic BP) and pulse pressure.

Other causes of hypovolaemic shock are listed in Table 6.1 (pages 105–6) and include a variety of clinical conditions associated with acute loss of blood, plasma or extracellular fluid. Patients with diarrhoea and vomiting, fever and dehydration all experience fluid loss associated with loss of body fluids. Patients with severe burns experience loss of body fluids and plasma, and this is explained in more detail in Chapter 10. Patients who experience third space fluid shift movements experience loss of fluid available to support the circulation. Fluid shifts into a space where it would not normally collect in such large volumes, such as with peritonitis, when fluid shifts into the peritoneal cavity, and with pancreatitis and ileus, when fluid shifts into the gastro-intestinal cavity (Redden and Wotton 2002a, 2002b).

When assessing patients with a history of excessive fluid loss it is important to assess factors such as evidence of dehydration, including dry mucus membranes, dry furred tongue and sunken eyeballs. Clinical signs can determine the severity of the patient's condition and also the likely cause. Assessing and communicating all the clinical signs and information collated to the care team can improve the patient's potential for recovery and should be undertaken using a comprehensive and systematic approach recommended by the National Institute for Health and Clinical Excellence (NICE, 2007a) and illustrated in Chapter 1 (page 6).

Your role as a nurse in assessing, anticipating and interpreting the signs of a patient going into shock cannot be overestimated. The responsibility for assessing, interpreting, differentiating and communicating information is central to the effective management of these patients. The core assessment criteria you should use have been introduced in Chapter 1 and will be illustrated in patient examples in the remainder of the chapter.

The assessment and management of patients who have the potential to develop shock should, wherever possible, include knowledge of their recent and past medical and social history. The role of the nurse is to develop a holistic and empirical knowledge of the patient so that any influencing factors that increase the patient's risk of developing problems are highlighted and put into context. Using the case study of Terry Jones below, we will explore the nurse's role in assessing, recognising and managing a patient with hypovolaemic shock at each stage of shock, and the underpinning pathophysiology.

Initial stage of hypovolaemic shock

Case study: Terry Jones collapses

Terry Jones (35 years) is a coach driver. He smokes at least 20 cigarettes a day and enjoys several pints after his driving is over for the day. Terry works irregular hours and is away from home several nights a week; as a consequence he tends to eat takeaway meals that he admits are unhealthy; however, he argues that his weight hasn't increased since he adopted this lifestyle and he has remained at 70kg. He recently went to his GP with back and shoulder pain and has been prescribed naproxen 500mg twice a day for four weeks. Over the last week he has complained of epigastric tenderness and stomach pain when he is hungry. At 19.00 hours that evening he is enjoying a pint in the hotel when he feels unwell and collapses on the way to the toilet. He vomits a large volume of brown liquid that looks as though it contains coffee granules (a potential clinical sign of altered blood). The paramedics estimate a fluid loss of at least 500 mls. Following an emergency admission to casualty he is admitted to a medical ward for assessment and management of a suspected gastric ulcer. He is assessed by the medical team as having a low risk of a further bleed and an endoscopy is booked for the following afternoon.

The nurse assesses Terry's condition at 21.30 hours using 'Look: Listen: Feel: Measure'. She finds that:

- *he is pale and cool to touch;*
- *he says he feels weak and sickly but thirsty for a cold drink of water;*
- *his respiratory rate is 18/min and regular;*
- *his pulse is 90/min and regular;*
- *his blood pressure is 100/65;*
- *his oxygen saturation is 95%;*
- *he is complaining of a dull ache in his abdomen and has a pain score of 4 out of 10 on a simple numerical scale (McCaffery and Beebe, 1993);*
- *he has not vomited since his collapse in the hotel or passed urine.*

Terry is demonstrating initial signs of shock (pale and cool, thirsty, and vital signs on the border of risk), and in spite of a fluid loss of approximately 10–12% he is able to maintain adequate circulation and perfusion. His body has been able to achieve this by triggering a response to hypovolaemic shock. The mechanisms involved in the body's response to shock include neural, chemical and hormonal compensation. In the sections below each of these is explained, but in reality these mechanisms are dynamic and interrelated in the process of returning the body to homeostasis.

Risk assessment, pathophysiology and priorities of care for initial stage

In the initial stages of shock patients' physiological responses are influenced by a number of factors. These include the cause and severity of the stressor or trauma (trigger/cause), the age of the patient and their general state of health. For example, the physiological effects of ageing can impact negatively on skin integrity, the musculoskeletal system and immune system; this leads to an increased risk of the patient having multiple pathologies and increased susceptibility to the effects of shock as in Megan's case (Watson, 2008). In Terry's case, following an assessment the medical team concluded that he was not in immediate danger as there were no signs of fresh blood loss, his vital signs were within acceptable parameters and he was young and otherwise healthy.

In the initial stage, any reduction in the volume of circulating blood is detected by pressure-sensitive baroreceptors and chemoreceptors sensitive to changes in carbon dioxide and oxygen in the arterial circulation, located in the arch of the aorta and carotid sinuses. When these receptors are triggered, impulses are relayed to the respiratory and cardiovascular centre in the medulla oblongata (brain stem), where they effect changes via the sympathetic nervous system to increase the pulse and force of cardiac contraction, trigger peripheral vasoconstriction and improve blood pressure. This trigger mechanism is illustrated in Figure 6.1.

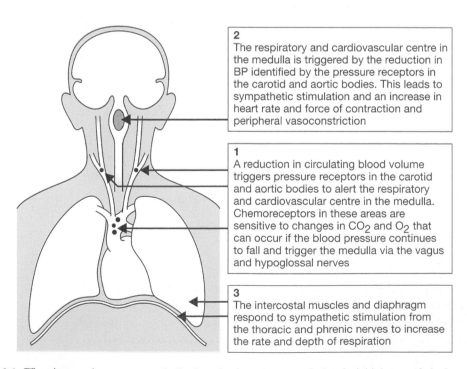

2
The respiratory and cardiovascular centre in the medulla is triggered by the reduction in BP identified by the pressure receptors in the carotid and aortic bodies. This leads to sympathetic stimulation and an increase in heart rate and force of contraction and peripheral vasoconstriction

1
A reduction in circulating blood volume triggers pressure receptors in the carotid and aortic bodies to alert the respiratory and cardiovascular centre in the medulla. Chemoreceptors in these areas are sensitive to changes in CO_2 and O_2 that can occur if the blood pressure continues to fall and trigger the medulla via the vagus and hypoglossal nerves

3
The intercostal muscles and diaphragm respond to sympathetic stimulation from the thoracic and phrenic nerves to increase the rate and depth of respiration

Figure 6.1: The trigger and compensatory feedback mechanisms that occur during the initial stage of shock

In Terry's case he is pale and cool to touch, suggesting evidence of vasoconstriction of the peripheral circulatory system. As a consequence, Terry's pulse and blood pressure are within the accepted range on the track and trigger score, and the priority for Terry is to identify and stabilise the cause of his condition and provide fluid replacement.

The key to successful management of patients in hypovolaemic shock is the assessment and early detection of the problem, followed by action to prevent or reduce further fluid loss. The primary aim is to restore clinically effective circulating volume while attempting to prevent further fluid loss. Fluid resuscitation of patients in hypovolaemic shock is complex and determined by a number of factors that relate to the patient and the primary cause. These include:

- the primary cause and type of fluid lost: blood, plasma, interstitial fluid;
- the age of the patient;
- evidence of co-morbidities such as heart failure, diabetes;
- fluid and electrolyte balance;
- blood glucose.

Case study: the management of Terry's condition at initial stage

An infusion of dextrose saline is commenced at a rate of 125ml/hour, ensuring that Terry's fluid intake is three litres per day to maintain hydration. He is to continue with nothing by mouth in order to rest the stomach and duodenum and promote healing. He has blood samples taken for a full blood count, blood group and cross match (in case of further bleeding), and to check urea and electrolytes and liver function. By 22.30 Terry is more comfortable and ready for sleep.

Terry continues to be at risk of further bleeding. However, because of his age (35 years), lack of co-morbidities, normal liver function and lack of evidence of clotting disorders, the risk is low. Terry needs to be monitored hourly overnight or until his condition improves, and he is asked to call the nurse with his call button if he feels sick (nauseated) or unwell in the night. In order to promote sleep and rest Terry needs his respirations, pulse and blood pressure monitored discreetly unless there is any further evidence of deterioration.

Compensatory stage of hypovolaemic shock

Case study: Terry Jones's condition deteriorates

Later that night at 00.30 hours Terry wakes feeling nauseated. Within minutes he has vomited 400mls liquid that tests positive to blood and appears to contain a mixture of fresh and partially digested blood (coffee ground vomit). He also wants his bowels open and requests a bedpan. He passes 350mls of a dark liquid stool that tests positive to blood (melaena). The nurse assesses Terry's condition at 00.30 hours using 'Look: Listen: Feel: Measure'. She finds that:

- *he appears pale, peripherally cyanosed and cold to touch;*
- *he is agitated and appears frightened;*
- *his respiratory rate is 24/min and regular;*

continued ...

- *his pulse is 110/min and regular;*
- *his blood pressure is 85/58;*
- *his oxygen saturation is 90%;*
- *he has passed 150ml of urine since his collapse in the hotel five-and-a-half-hours before;*
- *his arterial blood gases are: pH: 7.40 (n = 7.35–7.45); PaO₂: 9.3kPa (n = 10.6–13.3); PaCO₂: 4.2kPa (n = 4.7–6.7); HCO₃: 22.0mmol/l (n = 25–30).*

Risk assessment, pathophysiology and priorities of care for compensatory stage

The early clinical evidence of compensatory mechanisms at work include changes in respiratory rate as a result of increased pulse, changes in skin pallor and temperature as a result of peripheral vasoconstriction, and changes in blood pressure. In Terry's case both his respiratory and heart rate (pulse) increased and his blood pressure have decreased. An estimation of urine output since 19.00 hours indicates that he has passed less that 30mls per hour, signifying oliguria (reduced urine output <0.5ml/kg/hr). These findings, along with a change in his behaviour, are identified as putting him at risk and leads to a diagnosis of hypovolaemic shock with Terry's physiological systems attempting to compensate for the loss of blood volume.

The physiological response that occurs during the compensatory stage is immediate and occurs when adrenergic neurotransmitters stimulate alpha and beta 1 and 2 receptors in the smooth muscle of arterioles, cardiac muscle and skeletal muscle to increase heart rate, cause peripheral vasoconstriction and improve blood pressure. Stimulation of the beta 2 receptors also triggers bronchodilation and an added potential to improve lung ventilation by increasing the rate and depth of respiration, as illustrated in Figure 6.1. The sympathetic nervous system also triggers the adrenal medulla of the adrenal gland to release the catecholamines adrenaline and noradrenaline (epinephrine and norepinephrine) in order to continue providing the compensatory response, and this is illustrated in Figure 6.2. These are examples of negative feedback mechanisms that are used to restore homeostasis.

This stimulation of a sympathetic neural response occurs in most types of shock as part of the flight/fight response explained earlier. When an increase in heart rate and vasoconstriction does

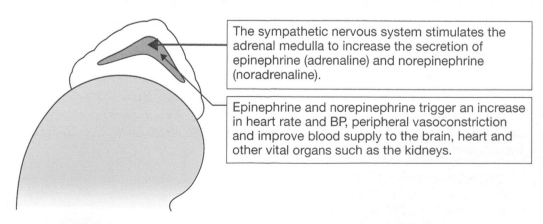

The sympathetic nervous system stimulates the adrenal medulla to increase the secretion of epinephrine (adrenaline) and norepinephrine (noradrenaline).

Epinephrine and norepinephrine trigger an increase in heart rate and BP, peripheral vasoconstriction and improve blood supply to the brain, heart and other vital organs such as the kidneys.

Figure 6.2: The triggering of the adrenal medulla that occurs during the compensatory stage of shock

not occur in the early stages of shock, this is usually due to one of two reasons. In neurogenic shock the sympathetic response may be impaired by spinal injury, nerve injury or drugs such as general anaesthetics (Mattson Porth and Matfin, 2009). In septic shock and anaphylactic shock the sympathetic response is challenged by a severe inflammatory response (Bridges and Dukes, 2005). Table 6.2 (pages 107–8) provides a comparison of the different features of shock found on clinical assessment and illustrates that the cause of shock can influence the early signs and symptoms.

The release of catecholamines, in the form of adrenaline (epinephrine) and noradrenaline (norepinephrine), continues to affect the alpha and beta receptors and thus continue the adrenergic response. The net effect of this is to influence respiratory rate and depth, increase heart rate, and improve blood flow to the coronary arteries, skeletal muscle, heart and brain through stimulation of the beta adrenergic receptors. The stimulation of alpha receptors continues to increase peripheral resistance by causing peripheral vasoconstriction, leading to coolness and pallor of the skin. Figures 6.1 and 6.2 illustrate the mechanisms involved in the initial and compensatory response, and Figure 6.3 illustrates the other mechanisms involved in providing physiological compensation (Mattson Porth and Matfin, 2009).

The initial fall in blood pressure also triggers a renal and a neural/adrenergic response. This response is described as the **renin-angiotensin-aldosterone mechanism**. Renin is an enzyme that is produced and stored in the juxtaglomerular cells of the kidneys. The juxtaglomerular cells are sensitive to changes in the responses of the sympathetic nervous system, and a reduction in blood flow to the kidneys will release renin into the circulation. Once in the circulation renin triggers the activation of **angiotensin I** from an inactive circulating protein. Angiotensin I is then converted by an enzyme called **angiotensin converting enzyme (ACE)** that is found in the lungs and kidney endothelial cells to **angiotensin II**, as the blood flows through the pulmonary circulation. Once activated, angiotensin II affects short- and long-term regulation of blood pressure.

- In short-term regulation, angiotensin II:
  - causes a vasoconstrictor effect on arterioles leading to increased peripheral vascular resistance and peripheral shutdown;
  - reduces sodium excretion from the kidneys so that the body retains more sodium and water.
- In long-term regulation, angiotensin II stimulates **aldosterone** secretion from the adrenal cortex. Aldosterone increases sodium and water retention by the kidneys. This increases the volume of extracellular fluid and circulating volume.

Another hormonal response triggered by reduced circulating volume and increased plasma **osmolarity** (increased concentration of salts) is **antidiuretic hormone (ADH)** or **vasopressin**. When triggered vasopressin is released from the posterior pituitary gland and has a powerful vasoconstrictor effect on arterioles in the systemic circulation. Vasopressin also has an antidiuretic effect and increases absorption of water from the kidneys in response to increased plasma osmolarity. These mechanisms are summarised in Figure 6.3.

For Terry this means that his peripheral temperature is cold, and there is evidence of peripheral shutdown from the peripheral cyanosis (blue-tinged nails on his hands and feet). The reduction in oxygen saturations suggests a reduction in perfusion and oxygenation of tissues due to loss of circulating blood volume, and the reduced urine output is indicative of the renin-angiotensin-aldersterone mechanism and antidiuretic hormone (vasopressin).

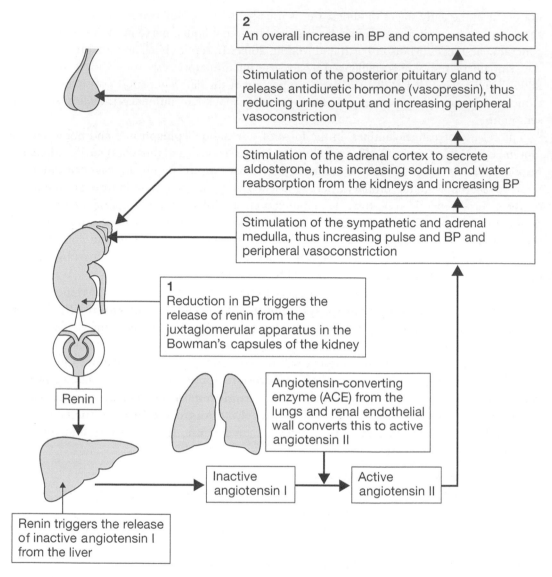

Figure 6.3: The compensatory mechanisms that occur as a physiological response to compensated shock

Case study: Management of Terry's condition at compensatory stage

Terry is considered to be at high risk, and the outreach team is called. Following an assessment of his condition, the outreach team commences the following treatment regime.

- *Fluid resuscitation commences with saline 0.9%, and a second intravenous access point is established for a transfusion of blood.*
- *High flow oxygen is commenced at 60%, and his oxygen saturations improves to 98%.*
- *Blood is taken for a full blood count (FBC) to determine his haemoglobin level (Hb), urea and electrolytes (U&E) to look for evidence of changes indicative of acute renal failure and an imbalance in electrolytes,*

continued . . .

> liver function tests (LFT), **prothrombin time (PT)** and **activated partial thromboplastin (APPT)** to assess for evidence of deranged clotting.
> - A urinary catheter is inserted and only 75mls of urine is collected, confirming oligurea.
> - An emergency endoscopy (a visual examination of the inside of Terry's stomach and duodenum), carried out once Terry is stabilised, reveals an actively bleeding peptic ulcer that is beginning to clot. It is agreed that Terry should be transferred to level 2 (high dependency care) for monitoring and stabilisation of his condition. He is commenced on a proton pump inhibitor (blocker) via the intravenous route to reduce gastric acidity and the risk of further bleeding, and he remains nothing by mouth. Proton pump inhibitors such as omeprazole block the production of stomach acid by shutting down a system in the stomach cells known as the proton pump, which is responsible for the production of stomach acid.

This is a critical point in Terry's care: his condition can either deteriorate or improve. In the following section two alternatives are provided for Terry's story.

- In the first story (Option 1), Terry's condition improves and he makes a full recovery.
- In the second story (Option 2), Terry's condition deteriorates and he becomes critically ill and goes into progressive shock.

Case study: Option 1 Terry Jones's condition improves

During the first night of Terry's admission to the high dependency unit his condition begins to stabilise and by the morning has improved. The nurse assesses Terry's condition at 08.00 using 'Look: Listen: Feel: Measure'. She finds that:

- *he looks pale, but his hands and feet are warm to touch and he feels tired but better;*
- *his respiratory rate is 14/min and regular (n = 12–20/min);*
- *his pulse is 80/min and regular (n = 60–80/min);*
- *his blood pressure is 120/72 (n = 100–140/60–90mmHg);*
- *his oxygen saturation is 98% (n = 95–100%);*
- *his arterial blood gases are: pH: 7.4 (n = 7.35–7.45); PaO_2: 14.3kPa (n = 10.6–13.3); $PaCO_2$: 4.7kPa (n = 4.7–6.7); HCO_3: 22.5mmol/l (n = 25–30);*
- *he has received fluid resuscitation with saline and blood and is now in a positive balance of two litres, with an average urine output of 80mls per hour.*

Risk assessment, pathophysiology and priorities of care during recovery from progressive stage (Option 1)

In this scenario option the improvement in Terry's condition following his episode of haematemesis and melaena suggest that his peptic ulcer is no longer actively bleeding and that the blood clotting seen on endoscopy has led to his condition stabilising. This improvement is evidenced by the improvement in his peripheral circulation – he is no longer cold and pale or peripherally cyanosed. He no longer feels anxious, and his vital signs are within the normal range. Terry shows no sign of a respiratory or metabolic acidosis, and his PaO_2 is higher than the normal range. As a result, Terry's oxygen is reduced to 40% and he is encouraged to drink clear fluids. Terry is also advised to avoid drugs such as naproxen, which is part of a group of **non-steroidal anti-inflammatory drugs** (NSAIDs) that are associated with an increased risk of gastric bleeding.

Activity 6.2   *Decision-making*

Terry has improved and his degree of risk has reduced.

1. How frequently would you assess his vital signs now that he is feeling better?
2. What clinical signs would indicate that Terry's condition was getting worse?
3. What information would you give Terry at this stage about his condition?

There are answers to this activity at the end of the chapter.

Progressive stage of hypovolaemic shock

Case study: Option 2 Terry Jones's condition deteriorates

During the first night of Terry's admission to the high dependency unit his condition continues to deteriorate. The nurse assesses Terry's condition at 04.00 using 'Look: Listen: Feel: Measure'. She finds that:

- *he still looks pale, peripherally cyanosed and cold to touch;*
- *he is confused and drowsy;*
- *his respiratory rate is 28/min with fast shallow respirations;*
- *his pulse is 120/min, sinus tachycardia;*
- *his blood pressure is 70/48;*
- *his oxygen saturation is 88%;*
- *he has passed 25–30 ml/hr since admission;*
- *his arterial blood gases are: pH: 7.23 (n = 7.35–7.45); PaO_2: 7.8kPa (n = 10.6–13.3); $PaCO_2$: 3.8kPa (n = 4.7–6.7); HCO_3: 15.5mmol/l (n = 25–30);*
- *urea is 11.5mmol/l (n = 2.5–6.5);*
- *creatinine is 155µmol/l (n = 55–105);*
- *lactate is 4.0mmol/l (n = 0.5–2.0).*

Risk assessment, pathophysiology and priorities of care for progressive stage (Option 2)

The clinical evidence suggests that Terry is going into type I respiratory failure (see Chapter 2). The clinical signs for this include confusion and drowsiness, increased respiratory rate accompanied by oxygen saturations (SaO_2) of less than 90% and partial pressure of arterial oxygen (PaO_2) levels of less than 8kPa (O'Driscoll et al., 2008).

Terry also has clinical evidence of a metabolic acidosis indicated by the reduced level of pH and bicarbonate in his arterial blood sample. The critical care team concludes that Terry has developed type I respiratory failure secondary to acute renal failure and a metabolic acidosis. The primary cause for his condition is shock induced by a severe gastro-intestinal bleed leading to inadequate tissue perfusion of vital organs such as the brain, leading to confusion and drowsiness, and the kidneys, leading to acute renal failure and the development of progressive shock.

The compensatory mechanisms (during compensatory shock) that the body recruits are short-term measures to maintain circulation. As the period of time lengthens between the initiation of shock and its resolution, the patient moves to the progressive stage of shock as the compensatory mechanisms become detrimental to the patient in a number of ways.

1. Intense vasoconstriction causes a reduction in the perfusion of tissues and reduced access to oxygen leading to ischaemia. Terry is peripherally cold and showing signs of peripheral cyanosis.
2. With a marked reduction in oxygen, cells are starved of **adenosine triphosphate (ATP)** production through the aerobic pathway and lack the energy to function effectively.
3. The cells have to rely on a less efficient process of energy production through the anaerobic pathway that produces about 20% of the energy that is normally acquired though aerobic metabolism.
4. The anaerobic pathway produces lactic acid as a by-product of metabolism and this leads to increased acidity in cells and a lactic acidosis. This is evidenced by a raised lactate level and a metabolic acidosis. Terry's respiratory effort has increased in response to the metabolic acidosis in an attempt to compensate for the acidity of the blood. By increasing his respiratory rate Terry is breathing out more carbon dioxide and water in an attempt to eliminate hydrogen ions (a measure of acidity, see Chapter 2, pages 47–8).
5. The inflammatory response is triggered as a result of the ischaemia and damage caused by anaerobic metabolism. As a consequence, tissues in body organs become damaged and inflamed, leading to an increased risk of acute respiratory distress and impaired renal function.
6. Without energy the normal cell function cannot be maintained, and the cells swell due to the failure of the sodium/potassium pump to maintain the fluid balance inside the cell and increased cell permeability.
7. As shock progresses, the inflammatory mediators **histamine** and **bradykinin** exert their vasodilatory properties, leading to progressive hypotension and cellular hypoxia (insufficient supply of oxygen). For Terry this means that the longer he stays in the progressive stage of shock the greater the risk of his body organs failing.
8. Prolonged hypoxia leads to suppression of the sympathetic nervous response and the cardiac and respiratory centre in the medulla oblongata; as a result, the patient's level of consciousness deteriorates. If Terry's condition continues to deteriorate, he will become drowsier and lose consciousness.

As the shock becomes more progressive, tachypnoea, tachycardia and hypotension will persist, but there will also be evidence of system failure in the form of pulmonary and peripheral oedema, respiratory failure and renal failure manifested by increased demand for oxygen, central and peripheral cyanosis, decreased urinary output and confusion. There may also be evidence of paralytic ileus (absence of bowel sounds) and abdominal distension. The patient will have a metabolic acidosis and altered blood clotting as a result of the hypoxia and inflammatory response (Migliozzi, 2009). In Terry's situation the critical care team was aware of the potential for this and continued to monitor his vital signs, U&Es, clotting and arterial bloods gases, as well as provide respiratory, circulatory and nutritional support.

The extent of cellular and organ damage that occurs in this progressive stage of shock is determined by the severity of the cause and the period of time your patient spends in the progressive stage. If not reversed, this stage will lead to your patient developing overwhelming cellular damage and destruction, leading to the failure of organs and systems. At this stage the progress of shock becomes irreversible, their body will be unable to respond to supportive therapy and death is inevitable. In Terry's situation, due to the rapid risk assessment, his age and general fitness there is a good chance that the critical care team can assist in stopping his progression to refractory shock and he should recover.

Case study: Management of Terry's condition as he moves from the compensatory to the progressive stage of shock

Terry's condition is now critical, and as a result the team decides to increase respiratory support by intubation and ventilation with biphasic respiratory support (see Chapter 3), continue with fluid resuscitation and risk assess for evidence of sepsis (see Chapter 7). If his renal output doesn't improve by morning, the team will reassess for the initiation of renal replacement therapy to support Terry's failing kidney function.

Risk assessment, preventing refractory shock (Option 2)

Refractory shock could occur in Terry's case if the critical care team is unable to prevent the progression of cellular and tissue damage that will ultimately lead to irreversible failure of the respiratory, cardiovascular, hepatic and renal system. It is the effect of decreased oxygenation and nutrition, the inflammatory response and the release of toxins from ischaemic tissue that leads to refractory shock (Hall, 2011). In severe and/or prolonged shock the body is no longer able to compensate for the loss of circulating volume through the negative feedback systems illustrated in Figures 6.1, 6.2 and 6.3 and, instead, reaches a stage where an increase in the degree of shock causes a further increase in the degree of shock (a type of positive feedback) and any supportive therapy becomes incapable of saving a person's life. The priority is always to risk assess patients using the assessment strategies included in this chapter and to prevent the progression of shock before refractory shock can occur.

We have identified the importance of timing, rapid and accurate risk assessment and communication when caring for patients in shock. In the activity below you have an opportunity to practise risk assessment and decision making.

Activity 6.3   *Decision-making*

In your bay you have two patients causing concern.

Mrs Thompson was admitted for day surgery but was later admitted to your surgical ward following a history of post-operative nausea and vomiting. Her nausea and vomiting have continued for 12 hours, with limited relief from anti-emetic medication. The surgical team are reluctant to commence any supportive care such as an infusion, assuming that the patient's nausea will settle with the medication.

Mrs Jacks has not passed urine since her return from theatre six hours ago following a **laparoscopic cholecystectomy**.

1. What would you look for when undertaking a risk assessment of Mrs Thompson?
2. What would you look for when undertaking a risk assessment of Mrs Jacks?
3. What information would you collect before informing the medical team of any concerns you have?

There are sample answers for this activity at the end of the chapter.

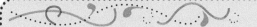

Chapter summary

The aim of this chapter was to help you to assess, recognise and respond to patients who go into shock. We have focused on the assessment and management of patients in hypovolaemic shock. In all of the clinical examples illustrated, the key responsibilities of the nurse are the same. They include the following.

- Carry out holistic assessment and monitoring of your patients.
- Know your patients and notice when the situation changes, even when the change is small.
- Ensure timely diagnosis and reporting of changes in the patient's condition: time is of the essence. Any patient who shows a change in their condition that is indicative of hypovolaemic, cardiogenic, obstructive or distributive shock should be risk assessed.
- Ensure there is continual monitoring and reporting of the patient's condition to the appropriate team.
- If unsure, act and express concern about your patient rather than hesitate and lose valuable time.

In Chapter 7 we continue to focus on assessing, recognising and responding to patients who go into shock, and we discuss the priorities of assessment and screening patients for sepsis and septic shock.

Activities: brief outline answers

Activity 6.2: Decision-making (page 120)

1. As Terry has improved and has appeared to stabilise, it is acceptable to reduce the frequency of observations from hourly to two hourly for four hours and, if he continues to improve, then reduce observations to every four hours. However, if you notice any change in his condition, you should review and risk assess. If you are concerned, increase the frequency of observation and communicate your concern according to the track and trigger score.
2. Look: Listen: Feel: Measure: the patient is pale, cool to touch, anxious; has increased respiratory rate, increased heart rate and reduced blood pressure; the patient is complaining of nausea, vomiting, diarrhoea, haematemesis and melaena.
3. At this stage in Terry's condition it is important to ask him what he understands about what has happened and explain what has happened and why. He will need reassurance that he is being monitored and being given treatment to promote healing and recovery. You should advise Terry to contact the nurse on the ward should he feel nauseated, unwell, faint or wanting to have his bowels open. These are all signs that the ulcer may be actively bleeding.

Activity 6.3: Decision-making (page 122)

1. Mrs Thompson has undergone minor surgery but has received nothing by mouth for an estimated 24 hours. She was probably asked to starve from midnight the night before her admission for minor surgery and has been suffering from nausea and vomiting ever since. She is in danger of developing hypovolaemic shock associated with dehydration. You need to assess the following using ABCDE and 'Look: Listen: Feel: Measure'.
   - Look, listen, feel for signs of dehydration: dry mouth, sunken eyes, thirst, anxiety, confusion, cool skin, evidence of pain.

- Measure: respiratory rate, pulse, BP, urine output and loss through vomiting, signs of negative fluid balance, time period without fluid intake and evidence of improvement following treatment with anti-emetic medication. Is there evidence of tachypnoea, tachycardia, and hypotension? What is the local track and trigger score?

Mrs Thompson is dehydrated and this is evidenced by tachypnoea, tachycardia and hypotension (respirations: 24, pulse: 98, BP: 88/58. She is reviewed based on the nurse's assessment and communication of findings and commenced on an intravenous infusion; she receives a fluid challenge of 500mls of 0.9% saline in 15 minutes, following which Mrs Thompson's vital signs improve to: respirations: 18; pulse: 90; BP: 95/58. She continues on 125ml/hour of intravenous saline and is encouraged to drink oral fluids as her nausea begins to subside. She feels much better the following morning and is discharged home that afternoon.

2. Mrs Jacks has not passed urine in the six hours post-operation. There could be a simple explanation in that no one has asked her or helped her to perform this activity. It could also be related to dehydration/ blood or fluid loss, or post-operative pain. You need to assess the following using ABCDE and 'Look: Listen: Feel: Measure'.

- Look, listen and feel for signs of blood/fluid loss and/or dehydration: dry mouth, sunken eyes, thirst, anxiety, cool skin, evidence of pain.
- Measure: respiratory rate, pulse, BP, urine output and loss through vomiting, signs of negative fluid balance, time period without fluid intake. Is there evidence of tachypnoea, tachycardia and hypotension?

Following an assessment of her condition Mrs Jacks reveals that she wants to pass urine but was too afraid to ask because everyone looked so busy! After some support and nursing care this patient is able to pass urine and begins to feel much more comfortable. Her vital signs are within the normal range and her pain is well managed.

3. Using SBAR you would collate the information you have collected above into:
   - the *situation*: reason for your call;
   - the clinical *background*: reason for patient's admission;
   - the changes that have occurred in the patient *assessment*: now or over time;
   - your *recommendation*: what you want the clinical team to do.

The patient causing concern was Mrs Thompson, and your prompt review has prevented this patient's condition from deteriorating and going into hypovolaemic shock.

Further reading

Edwards, S and Sabato, M (2009) *A nurse's survival guide to critical care.* Edinburgh: Churchill Livingstone.

This textbook provides a pocket-sized reference for practical aspects of caring for patients in critical care settings and provides factual and accessible information.

Higgins, C (2007) *Understanding laboratory investigations for nurses and health care professionals*, 2nd edition. London: Blackwell Publishing.

This textbook provides a user friendly approach to understanding laboratory investigations.

Moore, T and Woodrow, P (2009) *High dependency nursing care: observation, intervention and support for level 2 patients*, 2nd edition. London: Routledge.

This textbook focuses specifically on the care of level 2 patients and adopts a systematic approach to managing body systems.

Useful websites

www.mapofmedicine.com/

The mapofmedicine® site provides evidence-based multidisciplinary care maps of patients in diagnostic related groups and includes references to patients with medical and surgical problems as they undertake their journey through health care. The map is currently being used by 150 NHS organisations across England and Wales.

www.youtube.com/watch?v=4OcrG5eJO_0

This site provides a series of YouTube videos on shock that explore the details of changes in a patient's clinical signs and symptoms and clinical management.

Chapter 7
The patient with sepsis and distributive shock

Desiree Tait with Sandra Miles

Chapter aims

By the end of this chapter, you should be able to:

*   describe sepsis, severe sepsis, septic shock and systemic inflammatory response syndrome (SIRS);

- demonstrate an understanding of the causes of sepsis and severe sepsis;
- demonstrate an awareness of how to risk assess for sepsis and severe sepsis;
- demonstrate an awareness of the importance of managing blood pressure and circulation in the patient with severe sepsis and septic shock;
- reflect on the clinical examples used in the chapter and how they apply to your own experiences in practice.

Introduction

Case study: Mary's story

I have been working as a nurse in the community for two years now, and I have been visiting Tom to change the dressings on his leg ulcers once or twice a week for the last three months. Tom Parkin is 78 years old and has lived alone since his wife died of cancer a year ago. Since his wife's death, Tom has relied on the milkman to deliver his groceries, and he has avoided going out unless absolutely necessary. He has complained of venous leg ulcers on both legs for eight months and during the last three months there has been no change in their size or any evidence of healing. Last Friday I called in to change Tom's dressings and I noticed that Tom's left leg was more swollen than usual and the skin was hot and red. I was in a hurry and didn't check his vital signs, but I did make a mental note to call to see him on Monday just to check and take a wound swab if necessary.

When Monday came I didn't get to call on Tom until late afternoon, and when I did call there was no answer. I was an official key holder so I opened the key safe and let myself in. I found Tom breathless and disorientated; he said that he had fallen on the floor and been in the chair all weekend. He was hot to touch and his temperature with a tympanic thermometer was 39° C, R 40/min and pulse 100/min. I contacted the on-call GP, and Tom was subsequently admitted to the medical admissions unit later that evening. He was diagnosed with sepsis and dehydration. The GP congratulated me and said that if I hadn't visited that day Tom could have been a lot worse. However, I felt troubled.

- *Had I been too rushed last week?*
- *Had I missed vital clues?*
- *Should I have seen this coming?*
- *What could I have done that was different?*

When Mary phoned the ward on Tuesday she was informed that Tom had deteriorated further overnight and was now in ICU after being diagnosed with acute respiratory failure and severe sepsis. Tom required mechanical invasive ventilation (MIV) for five days and stayed in ICU for a total of seven days, after which he required acute care and rehabilitation for a further three weeks before being discharged home. Could Mary have risk assessed Tom's situation differently on Friday? Would it have made a difference to the outcome of his care? In the following sections we will explore how sepsis is defined, who is at risk and why. We will look back on Mary and Tom's story and explore how to risk assess for sepsis and severe sepsis in order to answer Mary's concerns.

What is sepsis?

An infection occurs when the body has been exposed to pathogenic organisms that have invaded and damaged body tissues. The body is able to recognise harmful invaders and provide a defence against the attack, containing and destroying the invader. This process is called the inflammatory response, and when it occurs locally in a particular body region – e.g. a tooth abscess, wound infection, a urinary tract infection – it can be contained and managed by the body's immune system. This is described as uncomplicated sepsis. In some instances this process requires the help of prescribed antibiotic therapy in order to assist the body in defending itself. For the majority of people the infection will be resolved without hospitalisation, and the patient will make a full recovery. For some patients, however, the disease can progress from an infection to sepsis (blood poisoning/septicaemia) and severe sepsis – the body's response to severe infection.

Sepsis can be described as the systemic inflammatory response to a recognised infection (Patrozou and Opal, 2010). Sepsis is associated with a syndrome known as systemic inflammatory response syndrome (SIRS), which occurs when we trigger a non-specific inflammatory response to an insult on the body. In the case of sepsis the insult is infection. However, it is important to recognise that other insults are also likely to lead to SIRS and these include:

- mechanical invasive ventilation (MIV);
- aspiration;
- major surgery;
- burns;
- pancreatitis;
- trauma.

Systemic inflammatory response syndrome is therefore associated with any situation that places severe trauma or stress on the body, including sepsis and severe sepsis. The relationship between sepsis and SIRS is illustrated in Figure 7.1.

The progression from sepsis to severe sepsis and septic shock can take several hours or several days. Severe sepsis can be life-threatening and is described as a clinical emergency. It is associated with a systemic inflammatory response and the dysfunction of at least one body system, which could be, for example:

- respiratory;
- cardiovascular;
- renal;
- hepatic;
- haematological;
- central nervous;
- metabolic acidosis that cannot be explained by other causes.

Severe sepsis can also be complicated by 'septic shock', and this is defined as severe sepsis with hypotension that has not responded to fluid resuscitation (Levy et al., 2003). Table 7.1 illustrates the clinical definitions of these terms and provides clinical examples of patients with those conditions.

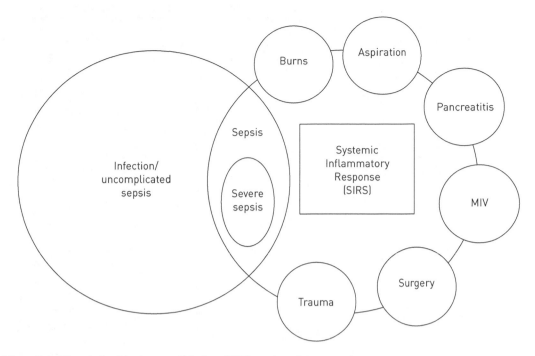

Figure 7.1: The relationships between infection, SIRS, sepsis and severe sepsis

Source: adapted from Bone et al. (1992).

Who is at risk and why?

In England, Wales and Northern Ireland the incidence of severe sepsis treated in hospital per 100,000 people increased from 46 in 1996 to 66 in 2003. The associated mortality rate from severe sepsis per 100,000 people also increased from 23 to 30 (Harrison et al., 2006). According to the International Sepsis Forum (2003), the incidence of sepsis has increased internationally over time and particularly in hospital patients as a result of the following.

- The use of invasive medical and technological interventions associated with treatments.
- The increasing number of older patients with co-morbidities (multiple disorders).
- The widespread use of antibiotics, which has led to an increasing incidence of drug-resistant micro-organisms.

Individuals who are most at risk of developing sepsis are:

- the very young and the very old, who are more likely to be immuno-compromised;
- patients with a weakened immune system due to treatments such as immuno-suppressant drugs used in inflammatory disorders and cancer treatment;
- patients with traumatic injuries;
- patients with addictions such as alcohol, smoking and drugs who potentially are already immuno-compromised or have damaged organs;
- patients who have invasive interventions such as intravenous catheters, urinary catheters, mechanical invasive ventilation;
- patients who have a disorder that increases their risk of developing sepsis, such as cystic fibrosis or human immune deficiency (HIV).

Terminology	Definition	Clinical examples
Infection or uncomplicated sepsis	A local inflammatory response to pathogenic organisms that have invaded and damaged body tissues.	• Molly James has been complaining of toothache and a swollen hot left cheek for several days. A visit to the dentist confirmed the presence of a tooth abscess.
Systemic inflammatory response syndrome (SIRS)	A systemic inflammatory response to an insult that results in tissue damage such as infection, pancreatitis, burns, in the presence of at least two of the following: • Temperature >38°C or <36°C. • Heart rate (pulse) >90/min. • Respiratory rate>20/min or $PaCO_2$ <4.3kPa. • White blood cell count (WBC) >12 x10^9/l or <4 x10^9/l. • Acutely altered mental state. • Hyperglycaemia >7mmol/l in the absence of diabetes.	• Paul Smith was involved in a road traffic collision that resulted in him sustaining crush injuries to his chest and upper abdomen. Within 24 hours he had evidence of: • T: 38.5°C; • P: 98/min; • R: 36/min; This indicated clinical evidence of SIRS.
Sepsis	A systemic inflammatory response to a documented infection and the presence of at least two of the criteria for SIRS (listed above).	Tom Parkin in Molly's story has been diagnosed with sepsis (see page 127).
Severe sepsis	A diagnosis of sepsis accompanied by the failure of at least one body system such as: acute respiratory distress syndrome and respiratory failure (Chapter 3), acute tubular necrosis and renal failure.	Tom Parkin went on to develop severe sepsis. Henry Mason (see the scenario on p 140) has been diagnosed with severe sepsis secondary to a urinary tract infection and acute respiratory failure.
Septic shock	A diagnosis of severe sepsis with hypotension that cannot be corrected by fluid resuscitation.	Sarah Clark (aged 70 years) was admitted to the emergency unit with a two-day history of back and abdominal pain and vomiting. Sarah has chronic renal failure for which she receives dialysis twice a week. On assessment (Look: Listen: Feel: Measure):

Multiple organ dysfunction (MOD)	Severe sepsis may progress to the failure of more body systems leading to multiple organ failure. This progression may begin with respiratory failure and progress through cardiovascular failure, renal failure and liver failure. Mortality rate for patients with MOD is high.	• warm and flushed; • lethargic and drowsy; • T: 38.5°C; • P: 136/min; • R: 38/min; • SaO₂: 87% on 60% oxygen; • BP: 75/50 (fluid resuscitation failed); • urine output 10 ml/hr. Sarah is showing signs of septic shock accompanied by acute respiratory failure together with existing renal failure. James Green (38 years) was diagnosed as HIV positive ten years ago. He was admitted to ICU with pneumonia. Within 24 hours of admission James had the following problems: • deeply unconscious (GCS: 4); • T: 38.8°C; • P: 136/min; • R: respiratory support; • SaO₂: 80% on 100% oxygen; • BP: 75/50 (failed fluid resuscitation); • urine output 20ml/hr with elevated urea and creatinine levels. James is showing signs of septic shock and MOD, with evidence of respiratory, renal, neurological and cardiovascular failure.

Table 7.1: Patient examples and clinical definitions of sepsis

Patients can acquire sepsis outside hospital (community acquired); Tom Parkin, described in Mary's story (page 127), is an example. These patients are often less difficult to manage in a clinical setting because they have not been exposed to interventions and procedures likely to increase their risk of developing sepsis with resistant strains of micro-organisms (International Sepsis Forum, 2003).

Why was Tom Parkin at risk?

Looking back at Mary's story, there were a number of factors that would have increased Tom's risk of developing sepsis. These include:

- age (78 years);
- open wounds associated with the venous ulcers;
- reduced mobility and circulation;
- psychological stress and loneliness;
- loss of appetite and possible malnutrition due to an imbalanced diet.

Tom appeared to still be grieving for his wife and as a result he had taken to staying at home, existing on a diet of whatever he could order from the milkman and generally losing motivation. Tom's immune system was impaired by his age, stress and malnutrition. The risk of him developing sepsis, therefore, had increased over time.

Nosocomial sepsis

Patients can also acquire sepsis in hospital (nosocomial), as will be described in Henry Mason's story (page 40). Cases such as Henry's are often more difficult to manage than community-acquired sepsis because the patient is already sick, will have been exposed to invasive procedures, may have already been on antibiotics and may be exposed to resistant strains of infection that tend to occur in hospital settings (International Sepsis Forum, 2003).

Risk assessing for sepsis: what are we looking for?

Sepsis usually originates from a localised infection that leads into an uncontrolled systemic response (Identifying Sepsis Early Group, 2006). When risk assessment and sepsis screening are used to identify sepsis as soon as it begins to emerge and appropriate interventions are initiated, there is evidence that survival rates can improve and patients can be prevented from progressing to the more severe forms of the disease (Levy et al., 2010; Rivers et al., 2001).

1. *Sepsis*: As we have seen, sepsis is a systemic inflammatory response to a documented infection and the presence of at least two of the diagnosing criteria for SIRS. A screening tool for sepsis should therefore have guidance on how to assess for evidence of infection and SIRS. An example of how a screening tool might look is illustrated in Figure 7.2 and follows guidance from the 1000 Lives Plus campaign, NHS Wales (2010) and Daniels and Nutbeam (2009).
2. *Severe sepsis*: The progression from sepsis to severe sepsis can take place in a matter of hours. Therefore sepsis screening should not end with the initiation of evidence-based treatment for sepsis but should also include the continued risk assessment for severe sepsis (illustrated in Figure 7.2).

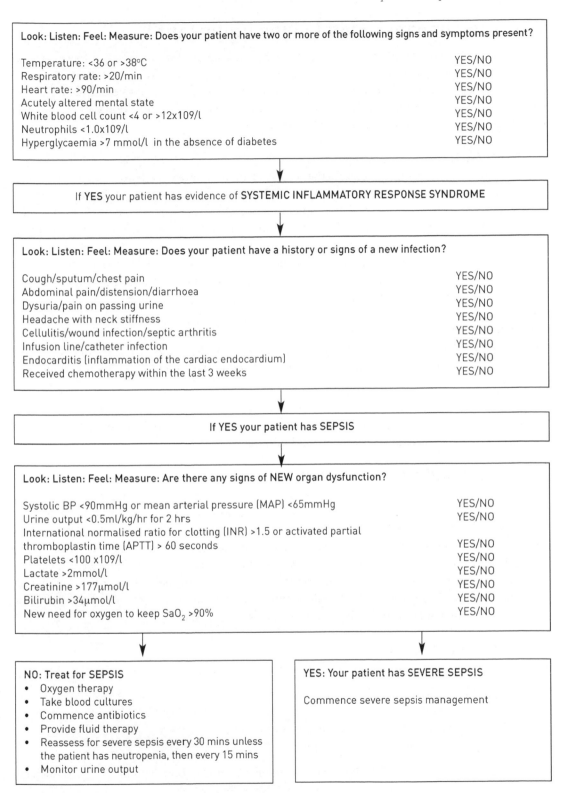

Figure 7.2: Sepsis and severe sepsis screening, a multidisciplinary assessment

Source: Adapted with permission from R. Daniels, Heart of England sepsis screening tool. Accessed at: www.survivingsepsis.org/SiteCollectionDocuments/Sepsis%203+3%20tool%20ward%20_2_.pdf.

Why are changes in vital signs important?

In this section we will explore in more detail the significance of clinical signs and focus particularly on temperature, respiration, heart rate, systolic blood pressure (SBP), mental state and signs of infection. Figure 7.3 provides a summary of the relationship between physiological factors and clinical signs, and Table 7.2 provides a summary of the clinical signs of infection for body systems most likely to be associated with the development of sepsis.

Temperature

A fever or pyrexia occurs in response to the release of inflammatory mediators or chemicals that trigger inflammation. These include cytokines and histamine, and are triggered by an event that causes damage to body tissues and cells, including infection (Hall, 2011). This process can be initiated within minutes or hours of damage by pathogens (infective organisms). Not all patients with sepsis or SIRS will present with pyrexia; exceptions include patients who have impaired temperature regulation such as patients with cervical spinal injury, people who are taking anti-inflammatory medication and patients where there is evidence of systemic inflammatory response but no evidence of infection.

Respiration

One of the earliest clinical signs of sepsis is an increase in the patient's respiratory rate. This increase may be triggered by a number of factors related to the patient's condition and include:

* pyrexia;
* evidence of respiratory infection or existing disease;
* pulmonary oedema triggered by a systemic inflammatory response leading to increased capillary permeability and leaking of fluid into the alveoli.

Heart rate and blood pressure

When a systemic inflammatory response is triggered, the flight/fight response (Chapter 6) is initiated, and the heart rate, cardiac output and blood pressure will initially increase in an attempt to compensate for changes that occur during the systemic inflammatory response. Key changes triggered by the release of inflammatory mediators include vasodilation, capillary leak, hypovolaemia and hypoxaemia. The body will try to maintain its homeostatic balance by drawing on fluid reserves in the liver, spleen and mesenteric circulation. If the inflammatory mediators continue unabated, however, the body will be unable to maintain a systolic blood pressure over 90mmHg and the patient will develop severe sepsis and septic shock.

Altered mental state

When a patient presents with an altered mental state, it can include a range of signs such as being:

* lethargic, sleepy, with disorganised movements;
* disorientated, restless;
* bewildered, having difficulty with obeying commands;
* stuporous (having reduced alertness), comatose.

In relation to sepsis and SIRS this altered state may be due to one or more of the following:

* hypoxia;
* hypovolaemia and electrolyte imbalance;
* damage to the neurological system as a direct result of sepsis.

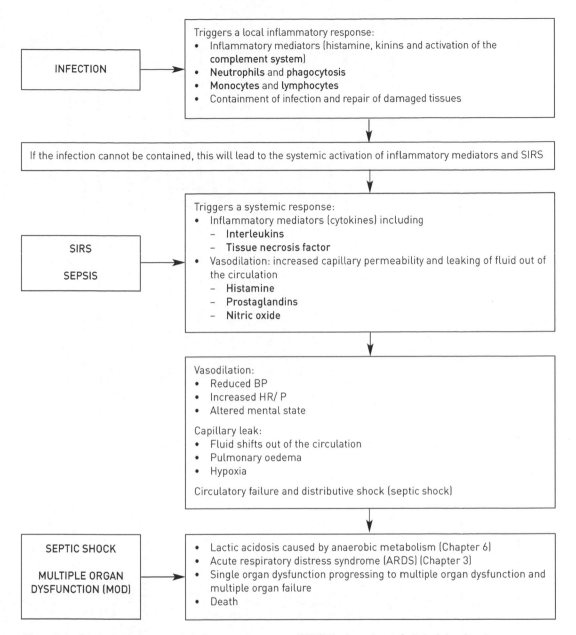

Figure 7.3: Sepsis: how the systemic inflammatory response (SIRS) leads to signs of clinical deterioration

Signs of infection

The changes in clinical signs, together with evidence of infection provide vital information when screening for sepsis or clinical deterioration. The most common sites for infection that are associated with the development of sepsis are:

- lungs;
- skin;
- abdomen;
- urinary tract.

The clinical signs of infection related to these sites are listed in Table 7.2.

Body system	Signs of infection: Look: Listen: Feel: Measure	Clinical examples
Lungs	• R: > 20/min. • Dyspnoea. • Temperature >38°C. • Yellow/green sputum when expectorating. • Noisy air entry during auscultation and/or no air entry to some lung quadrants. • Evidence of consolidation on chest X-ray.	Serena Jones (18 years) works in a busy city centre store. She has had a flu-like illness for eight days and still feels unwell. She returned to work because she is worried that too much time off would reflect badly on her record. Within an hour Serena collapsed on the floor while serving a customer; she was faint, breathless and exhausted. Her respirations were 28/min and her temperature is 38.8°C. Serena was diagnosed with pneumonia (see Chapter 3). *Serena recovered without developing sepsis.*
Skin	• Cellulitis: inflamed, red, hot and swollen area of skin that is spreading from a focal point. • Petechial rash (rash of blood spots). • Temperature >38°C. • Evidence of invasive catheterisation of the skin. • Wounds: pain, tenderness, inflammation, pus. • Characteristic smell.	Peter Matthews (70 years) has type II diabetes. A week ago he bought new shoes; unfortunately the shoes rubbed and he developed a blister on his left heel. Several days later he noticed his heel, ankle and foot were swollen and red. He made an appointment at the local surgery for the following day. By the time he was assessed by the doctor his leg was red, hot and inflamed up to his knee and he felt hot and tired. His temperature was 39°C. Peter was diagnosed with cellulitis and admitted for 24 hours' observation and intravenous antibiotic therapy. *Peter developed sepsis and required care in ICU.*
Abdomen	• Abdominal pain or tenderness. • Temperature >38°C. • Nausea/vomiting. • Diarrhoea.	Barry Andrews (74 years) enjoyed a party and buffet meal to celebrate his granddaughter's 18th birthday. Two days later he developed acute abdominal pain, nausea, diarrhoea and felt feverish with a temperature of 39.4°C. His symptoms continued for four days before he required admission to hospital for further management. He was diagnosed with a *campylobacter* infection. *Peter developed severe sepsis and septic shock and is still receiving intensive therapy.*
Urinary tract	• Cystitis/pain on passing urine (dysuria). • Frequency and/or urgency when passing urine. • Cloudy urine with a characteristic smell. • Haematuria.	Sandra Brown (17 years) is a first-year undergraduate at university. For the last week she has experienced frequency and urgency when passing urine. Today she awoke with pain in her right loin which increased in severity when she tried to pass urine. Sandra felt nauseated and shivery. She was advised during a visit to the campus medical centre that she had a urinary infection and was asked to provide a specimen of urine for sampling. *Sandra made a complete recovery; she did not develop sepsis.*

Table 7.2: Clinical signs of infection in body systems

As a nurse you have direct responsibility for assessing and monitoring the patient's condition, even when you may have delegated the task to others. Your role when risk assessing for sepsis includes the following activities.

- Adopting a patient-centred approach to care and knowing your patient.
- Risk assessment and monitoring of the patient using the principles of 'Look: Listen: Feel: Measure'.
- Effective communication and collaboration with the health care team.
- Effective use of clinical pathways and guidance to interpret, recognise and respond to clinical signs of deterioration in a timely manner.

Case study: Tom Parkin: what could Mary have done differently?

If we look back at Mary's story about Tom, a number of factors can be highlighted that, with hindsight, could have made a difference to Tom's care.

- *Adopting a patient-centred approach to care and knowing your patient were significant in Tom's case because of the evidence of the gradual decline identified in the risk assessment.*
- *Using risk assessment and monitoring the patient using the principles of 'Look: Listen: Feel: Measure' were also key factors. If Mary had risk assessed Tom on Friday when she noticed some changes in his condition she would have identified evidence of cellulitis and a wound infection. Assessment of his T, P, R and BP might have confirmed this, and a swab could have been sent earlier to identify the infecting organism (Scottish Intercollegiate Guidelines Network, 2010).*
- *Effective communication and collaboration with the health care team on Friday would have also alerted the team to the change and, at the least, an earlier review of Tom's condition.*
- *The effective use of clinical pathways and guidance to interpret and recognise clinical signs of deterioration is another factor. This process was not used on the Friday but was used 72 hours later on Monday afternoon when Tom's condition had deteriorated. Using the sepsis screening guide in Figure 7.2 we can see that he presented with the following evidence of systemic inflammatory response syndrome and sepsis.*
  - *Temperature: >38°C.*
  - *Respiratory rate: >20/min.*
  - *Heart rate: >90/min.*
  - *Altered mental state.*

Tom also presented with evidence of cellulitis in his left leg, which is indicative of infection.

By spending an extra 15 minutes with Tom on Friday, Mary could have risk assessed him for evidence of infection, SIRS and sepsis, and communicated her concerns to the general practitioner. This might have prevented him from developing sepsis, but if not, it would have ensured the initiation of sepsis screening earlier and the prevention of severe sepsis. By reflecting on her care, Mary could not change what happened to Tom but she can use this experience to improve her risk assessment and management of other patients in her care.

Activity 7.1 gives you an opportunity to practise assessing patients for evidence of sepsis.

Activity 7.1   *Decision-making*

With the aid of the sepsis screening tool in Figure 7.2 review the scenarios below and determine if any of the patients meet the criteria for either SIRS, sepsis or severe sepsis.

Edward Morris (69 years) has been diagnosed with inoperable carcinoma of the large bowel. This had been confirmed by a second laparoscopic bowel biopsy in two weeks as the first had proved inconclusive. Edward was commenced on chemotherapy one week later and completed the first 14-day cycle of treatment as an outpatient. Seven days later he began to experience acute abdominal pain in the right side of his abdomen and began to feel hot, shivery and unwell. The guidance on his chemotherapy care pathway directed him to monitor his temperature and contact the ward if his temperature was above 38°C. His temperature was 38.6°C and his pulse, taken by his daughter, was 95/min. He contacted the ward staff for advice.

1. Did Edward meet any of the screening criteria?
2. What advice would you give Edward?

Molly Taylor (73 years) has been admitted to an acute medical ward with a history of falls. On this occasion she had been found by the milkman who heard her calling for help through the bathroom window. She had got up to go to the toilet at 02.00 hours and had lost consciousness for several hours. Molly had not broken any bones, and apart from a bloodied nose, there appeared to be no clear reason for her loss of consciousness. Nine hours after admission she became short of breath and disorientated. Her daughter was visiting at the time and said that Molly did not normally suffer from confusion and that the only relevant thing that had happened in the last few weeks was they had all been suffering from a heavy cold and that Molly had taken to her bed for three days.

Using the principles of 'Look: Listen: Feel: Measure' Molly presented with:

- confusion;
- R: 28/min;
- P: 95/min;
- T: 37.9°C;
- BP: 100/60;
- SaO_2: 88%.
1. Did Molly meet any of the screening criteria?
2. How would you respond to Molly's condition?

There are answers to this activity at the end of the chapter.

What are the priorities of care for a patient diagnosed with sepsis?

So far in this chapter we have focused on risk assessment and diagnosis of a patient with sepsis. The next step is to assess the patient situation, which includes questioning whether there are any limitations of treatment that exist for your patient. Are these limitations still valid? It is important not to make assumptions about a patient's care and, if possible, always to involve the patient and family in the decision-making process (see Chapter 1).

When a patient is diagnosed with sepsis the speed of response is critical in order to prevent further deterioration. The Surviving Sepsis Campaign (SSC, 2011) recommends that resuscitation and diagnosis interventions should be initiated immediately, and it identifies a set of six tasks that should be completed within the first hour following recognition of sepsis.

This group of multidisciplinary interventions is called the 'Sepsis Six', and adopting this plan in a timely manner can reduce patient mortality by half (SSC, 2011). They include the following.

- *Give high flow oxygen* (via a non-rebreathing bag if appropriate): according to Daniels (2011) these patients should receive high levels of oxygen regardless of their underlying condition, although he recommends that patients with COPD should be managed by a specialist clinician.
- *Take blood cultures*: this should be completed before antibiotic therapy has commenced unless this is contraindicated. This is also the time to take samples and swabs of any likely source of infection if appropriate.
- *Give intravenous antibiotics*: the use of prescribed broad spectrum **empirical antibiotic therapy** can be initiated before the infecting organism is identified and reviewed when more information is available.
- *Start intravenous fluid resuscitation*: if the patient has a systolic BP of >90mmHg, a reasonable fluid prescription would include 500mls of Hartmann's solution to be administered over 30–60 minutes. If the patient has a systolic blood pressure of <90mmHg, then the patient should receive 20mls/kg/l of Hartmann's solution over 30–60 minutes.
- *Check blood levels of haemoglobin and lactate.*
  - A fall in the patient's blood haemoglobin below 7–9g/dl^{-1} can adversely affect patient outcome; the patient's haemoglobin should therefore be monitored in order to reduce this risk (Walsh and Ezz-El-Din Saleh, 2006).
  - A lactate level of >2mmol/l in patients with sepsis is indicative of anaerobic metabolism due to reduced tissue perfusion (shock), particularly if the high level persists over several days.
- *Accurately monitor hourly urine output*: if the patient does not have a urinary catheter inserted, then it is necessary to organise this. A urine output of <0.5ml/kg/hr for two hours is evidence of reduced perfusion to the kidneys (shock) and can lead to acute renal failure.

In the next scenario we will discuss the care of Henry Mason and examine how he was risk assessed and managed in the early hours of his change in condition.

Case study: Henry Mason

Henry is 71 years old. He used to smoke 20 cigarettes a day but gave up 20 years ago when he was diagnosed with type II diabetes. He has very poor eyesight due to bilateral cataracts and is waiting for surgery. He's had hypertension and been on medication for ten years. Henry has already been in hospital for a week. He was originally admitted with pneumonia, and following a respiratory arrest on the medical ward, he spent five days in ICU. During his stay in ICU he required MIV to support his respiratory function as well as intravenous antibiotic therapy, physiotherapy, haemodynamic and nutritional support. In order to monitor and support his condition he had an arterial line, a central line, a urinary catheter and intubation with an endotracheal tube. By the time Henry was discharged from ICU, he was breathing with the support of 40% oxygen, and his urinary catheter, central line and arterial line had been removed.

He was making good progress, but 48 hours after his discharge to the ward, Jan, the nurse looking after him, noted that he was reluctant to eat and drink, he was lethargic and his chest sounded noisy. Henry's respiratory rate had increased to 21/min from 18/min but otherwise his vital signs remained unchanged (T: 37.5°C; P: 89/min; BP: 130/85mmHg). Jan communicated her concerns to the medical team at 18.00 hours and recorded them in the notes.

Was Henry at risk of developing sepsis?

An examination of Henry's care plan showed that he was at high risk of developing sepsis for the following reasons.

- His age: 71 years.
- He has co-morbidities including diabetes, hypertension and recovering from pneumonia.
- He had required invasive lines and catheters to support his respiratory and cardiovascular function in ICU.
- He is on antibiotic therapy for pneumonia.

Activity 7.2	*Decision-making*

- With reference to the sepsis screening tool in Figure 7.2, can you identify if Henry met any of the criteria for SIRS and sepsis?
- Using the screening tool and the recognition and response bundles identified in Chapter 1 (Table 1.2), plan what you would do to support optimum management of Henry from 18.00 hours to 19.00 hours.

The answers are discussed later in the chapter in the case study 'Henry's care between 18.00 and 22.00 hours' on page 143.

When we return to Henry's care, nearly four hours have passed, and apart from reporting her concerns, Jan has done nothing more for Henry apart from sit him up in bed. She is preparing to hand over her concerns to the night staff.

Scenario: Henry Mason's condition deteriorates

By 22.00 hours when the night shift took over, Henry's condition had deteriorated further. Using 'Look: Listen: Feel: Measure', his assessment was as follows.

- *He was breathless and dyspnoeic and centrally cyanosed with SaO_2: 84.*
- *He was confused and working hard to breathe.*
- *He felt hot with dry skin*
- *T: 38.8°C.*
- *R: 30/min.*
- *P: 110/min.*
- *BP95/65 mmHg.*
- *He had not passed urine since 17.00, and this was recorded as 100ml of cloudy urine.*

Henry now met more than two of the criteria for SIRS and sepsis, with evidence of possible sites of infection in the lungs and urinary tract. John, the nurse on the night shift, contacted the critical care outreach team, communicating the information using the SBAR communication tool. He stayed with the patient and delegated a member of staff to collect and prepare the following.

- *A high flow oxygen mask.*
- *The equipment required for sampling of blood cultures and arterial sampling.*
- *A trolley set up for urinary catheterisation.*
- *Some infusion fluid (Hartmann's solution 1L).*

The next activity gives you an opportunity to practise what you would include in the SBAR document.

Activity 7.3   *Decision-making*

Using Table 1.8 (page 20) as a guide, identify the information you would include in the SBAR documentation when Henry deteriorated at 22.00.

The answer is given at the end of the chapter.

Henry's story continues in the next scenario, which illustrates how the 'Sepsis Six' bundle of interventions was used.

Scenario: Henry Mason is transferred to ICU

22.10 hours: *Within ten minutes the outreach team had arrived, and the 'Sepsis Six' interventions were commenced.*

- *High flow oxygen therapy.*
- *Blood cultures.*

continued . . .

- *Intravenous antibiotics.*
- *Blood samples including arterial blood gases, haemoglobin, urea, and electrolytes and lactate.*
- *Insertion of a urinary catheter.*
- *Fluid challenge of 500 ml of Hartmann's solution.*

After the fluid challenge Henry became increasingly breathless, and he was immediately transferred to ICU.

22.50 hours: When Henry was admitted to ICU he was intubated and ventilated using bilevel ventilation (inspiratory pressure: 25cm H20, expiratory pressure: 5cm H_2O) in order to support his failing respiratory function.

An assessment using 'Look: Listen: Feel: Measure' identified the following.

- *Unrousable after being given sedation to facilitate intubation.*
- *T: 38.8°C.*
- *R: 15/min set rate on the ventilator/no spontaneous respiration.*
- *P: 120/min.*
- *BP: 88/60mmHg.*

After being catheterised Henry had drained a reservoir of 50ml of cloudy urine since last collected at 17.00 hours; a catheter sample of urine was taken for culture and microscopy. A chest X-ray showed pulmonary oedema, and his arterial blood sample on admission with 90% oxygen was:

- *pH: 7.166;*
- *PaO_2: 7.8kPa;*
- *$PaCO_2$: 6.61kPa;*
- *HCO_3: 16.0;*
- *BE: −9.*

Other relevant blood results included:

- *haemoglobin (Hb): $9.7g/dl^{-1}$;*
- *lactate 5.6mmol/l;*
- *urea: 15mmol/l;*
- *creatinine: 245mmol/l;*
- *sodium (Na): 145mmol/l;*
- *potassium (K): 6mmol/l.*

23.00 hours: Henry was showing signs of severe sepsis and septic shock revealed by his:

- *hypoxia;*
- *reduced blood pressure;*
- *reduced urine output;*
- *high lactate level and metabolic acidosis.*

Henry was also showing signs of acute respiratory failure with evidence of hypoxia and pulmonary oedema, and acute renal failure with evidence of an increased urea and creatinine level and increased potassium level.

Henry is now critically ill and may not survive; in the case study box below we look back at his care at 18.00 hours and reflect on how this has impacted on his condition.

Case study: Henry's care between 18.00 and 22.00

If we look back at Henry's care between 18.00 and 22.00 hours there are a number of factors that led to a substantial delay in responding to his clinical deterioration.

- *Jan, the nurse looking after Henry on the late shift, had reported the change in his condition that at the time identified him as meeting the criteria for sepsis and SIRS. The response from the medical team, however, was to note it and not respond to the change.*
- *Jan should have continued monitoring the patient every 15 minutes and again contacted the medical team and the critical care outreach team to assess the patient, informing them that Henry met the criteria for sepsis and needed immediate assessment.*
- *If the 'Sepsis Six' interventions had been commenced at 18.00 hours instead of 22.00 hours, Henry's chances of survival would have significantly improved.*

When assessing and screening for sepsis, timing is critical and the nurse's role in assessing and communicating clinical information cannot be overestimated. If the incidence of severe sepsis is to be reduced, then every member of the health care team needs to work collaboratively and collectively to achieve that goal.

How should patients with severe sepsis be managed?

As we have seen, when a patient is diagnosed with sepsis/severe sepsis, it is important to involve the critical care outreach team and transfer the patient to ICU as soon as possible because these patients will need intensive support of their respiratory, cardiovascular and circulatory systems in order to support their body organs, prevent multiple organ dysfunction and improve their chances of survival. In the sections below we will explore how Henry was managed in relation to the Surviving Sepsis Campaign's international guidance on managing severe sepsis (SSC, 2011). This guidance recommends that the resuscitation and management bundles for patients with severe sepsis should be completed within 24 hours of diagnosis in order to improve survival. This was achieved for Henry, although the delay in the early stages of sepsis recognition did reduce his risk of survival.

Airway and breathing

For some patients pneumonia may be the primary cause of sepsis, but this is not the case for all patients. Henry's first admission to ICU was due to pneumonia, but his second admission with sepsis was associated with a urinary tract infection. Most patients who develop sepsis will also develop respiratory failure associated with the systemic inflammatory response and, as in Henry's case, will develop hypoxia, pulmonary oedema and increased respiratory rates (tachypnoea). The aim of management is to support the patient's respiratory function and reduce the risk of any further damage by:

- providing respiratory support in order to achieve PaO_2 at >8kPa;
- adhering to the ventilator bundle explained in Chapter 3;
- reducing the risk of ventilator associated injury (Chapter 3, Table 3.6).

Cardiac and circulatory system

Patients with sepsis and particularly septic shock have hypotension associated with capillary leak (Figure 7.3). The aims of cardiovascular support are to ensure the patient has accurate, safe and continuous monitoring of their heart rate, blood pressure (arterial line), **central venous pressure** (CVP), temperature and urinary catheter in order to manage their fluid requirements. Fluid requirements for patients in septic shock are high, and Henry's case was complicated by his diagnosis of acute renal failure. Within 24 hours Henry was commenced on renal replacement therapy for the management of his renal failure, and invasive respiratory support continued to support his lung function. Goals of early directed therapy for patients with severe sepsis include:

- CVP >8mmHg (>12mmHg if ventilated);
- systolic blood pressure >90mmHg (mean arterial pressure >65mmHg).

Fluid replacement should continue until the patient's systolic blood pressure is above 90mmHg. If, as in Henry's case, the blood pressure does not respond to the fluid challenge and/or the patient becomes increasingly breathless, then the next level of cardiovascular support is introduced.

This involves the commencement of a group of drugs known as positive inotropes, which work by increasing peripheral vasoconstriction and improving blood pressure; many of them occur naturally in the body. They include adrenaline (epinephrine) and noradrenaline (norepinephrine). As a rule these drugs are given intravenously via a central line as they cause peripheral vaso-constriction. They have a half-life of approximately one to two minutes and should not be turned off unless prescribed as the patient will react within minutes with rebound hypotension and bradycardia. It is important, therefore, to assess and monitor your patient's haemodynamic state carefully as these drugs have a virtually instant effect on the cardiac and circulatory system. Noradrenaline is the first drug of choice and is infused until the patient is able to maintain a blood pressure above systolic 90mmHg (65–85 mean arterial pressure).

Disability and exposure

It is important to assess and review the patient's mental state and level of consciousness hourly as this can be a sign of improvement or deterioration (Chapter 9). In order to reduce the risk of further infection and control existing infections, it is essential to continue with core interventions related to infection prevention and control. These include:

- hand washing;
- appropriate use of uniforms and personal protective equipment;
- safe disposal of sharps;
- aseptic procedure and adherence to bundles of care such as the central line bundles (IHI, 2011b);
- assessment for evidence of developing infection at infusion sites and catheters;
- isolation of patients with health-care related infection;
- vaccination of health care staff.

Henry spent a further two weeks in ICU and was transferred to a medical ward for rehabilitation. By this time Henry had experienced acute respiratory failure, cardiovascular failure and renal failure. By the time he was discharged from ICU, his multi-organ failure was resolving, he felt weak, tired and anxious, and was still very dependent on nursing staff for support. Unfortunately, Henry died four weeks later from cardiac failure secondary to severe sepsis.

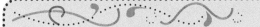

Chapter summary

The aim of this chapter was to help you to assess, recognise and respond in a timely manner to patients who develop sepsis and severe sepsis, including septic shock. The responsibilities of the nurse when caring for patients at risk of sepsis can be summarised as follows.

- Undertake a rigorous assessment and monitoring of the patients in your care.
- Know your patients and recognise that any change in their condition is significant.
- Use standard guidelines and protocols to support your decision making.
- Ensure that interventions are timely – they save lives; do not hesitate and lose valuable time.
- Report evidence of change or deterioration in the patient's condition to the relevant medical team and follow up your concerns.
- Anticipate and be prepared to support a patient's deteriorating condition.

Activities: brief outline answers

Activity 7.1: Decision-making (page 138)

Edward Morris:
1. Edward did meet some of the screening criteria and was clearly showing signs of sepsis.
   - T: 38.6°C.
   - P: 95/min.
   - Completed chemotherapy seven days ago.
2. Advice to give Edward.
   - Neutropenic sepsis is a medical emergency, so Edward should be advised to call 999 and ask for the ambulance service. Patients in Edward's situation need an urgent full blood count to determine if neutropenia is present.
   - While he is waiting he could collect his overnight bag and a summary of the chemotherapy drugs he has taken.

Molly Taylor:
1. Molly did meet some of the screening criteria and was showing signs of sepsis and hypoxia.
   - Confusion.
   - R: 28/min.
   - P: 95/min.
   - SaO$_2$: 88%.
2. Molly is in the high risk range of the response bundle (NICE, 2007a).
   - Using the SBAR framework, you should contact the outreach team and summarise Molly's current problems, background and most recent vital signs.
   - You should respond by anticipating the needs of the patient and outreach team when they arrive. While one person stays with the patient, someone can collect any equipment necessary as illustrated in Henry's story.

Activity 7.3: Decision-making (page 141)

Date and time of initial call: *22.00, 10/10/11* Date and time of response: *22.10, 10/10/11*	Patient's name: *Henry Mason: age 73 years* Nurse's name: *John James* Name of person called: *Outreach team*
Situation: Reason for the call	*I am concerned about Henry Mason. He was admitted two days ago from ICU. He was in ICU, ventilated for 5 days for management of pneumonia. He meets the criteria for severe sepsis and is in respiratory distress.*
Background	*He has type II diabetes and hypertension, previous smoker.*
Assessment	T: *38.8*; P: *110*; R: *30*; BP: *95/65*; oxygen saturations: *84%*; Blood glucose: *Not known.* Track and trigger score: *has increased.* Other relevant data: *Is for active resuscitation. Has been unwell for 4 hours. He is confused and dyspnoeic, centrally cyanosed, hot and flushed.*
Recommendations and response	What you are requesting: Ward visit*: Urgent.* Telephone advice:– Prescription: – Other: – • Action taken and Registrar's response: *Commence a high flow oxygen. I'll need equipment for blood cultures and arterial sampling, urinary catheterisation. Prepare an infusion of Hartmann's solution 1L.* Signatures: *Signed by both the staff nurse and the registrar following Henry's assessment.*

Table 7.3: Answer to Activity 7.3: the information to include in the SBAR documentation when Henry deteriorated at 22.00

Further reading

Daniels, R and Nutbeam, T (2009) *ABC of sepsis (ABC series)*. Oxford: Wiley-Blackwell.

This book offers a more detailed account of how patients with sepsis should be managed in acute and critical care areas and offers a pragmatic guide to the care of these patients.

Useful websites

www.ihi.org/explore/HAI/Pages/default.aspx

This website offers health care professionals information and practical advice on how to reduce health care associated infections and includes information on hand hygiene and reducing catheter-related urinary infections.

www.ncepod.org.uk/2008sact.htm

This site reports on a confidential inquiry into patient outcome and death following cancer chemotherapy and supports further reading for Activity 7.1: Edward Morris.

www.npsa.nhs.uk/cleanyourhands/resource-area/

This site is part of the National Patient Safety Agency website and offers information on hand hygiene and the 'Wi-five? Game'.

www.survivingsepsis.org/

This website offers information and advice on how to risk assess, resuscitate and manage patients with sepsis. It provides educational tools and updates on international guidelines for managing sepsis.

Chapter 8
The patient with acute confusion or delirium

Desiree Tait with Julie Wickland

NMC Standards for Pre-registration Nursing Education

This chapter will address the following competencies:

Domain 1: Professional values

1.1. Adult nurses must understand and apply current legislation to all service users, paying special attention to the protection of vulnerable people, including those with complex needs arising from ageing, cognitive impairment, long-term conditions and those approaching the end of life.

Domain 2: Communication and interpersonal skills

4. All nurses must recognise when people are anxious or in distress and respond effectively, using therapeutic principles, to promote their well-being, manage personal safety and resolve conflict. They must use effective communication strategies and negotiation techniques to achieve best outcomes, respecting the dignity and human rights of all concerned. They must know when to consult a third party and how to make referrals for advocacy, mediation or arbitration.

NMC Essential Skills Clusters

This chapter will address the following ESCs:

Cluster: Care, compassion and communication

2. People can trust the newly registered graduate nurse to engage in person-centred care empowering people to make choices about how their needs are met when they are unable to meet them for themselves.

By entry to the register:

x. Recognises situations and acts appropriately when a person's choice may compromise their safety or the safety of others.

xi. Uses strategies to manage situations where a person's wishes conflict with nursing interventions necessary for the person's safety.

Chapter aims

By the end of this chapter, you should be able to:

- describe the terms 'acute confusion' and 'delirium';
- identify the common causes of delirium;
- demonstrate an awareness of how to risk assess for and prevent delirium;
- demonstrate an awareness of how to manage patients with delirium and provide them with a safe environment;
- reflect on and practise the risk assessment and management of patients with delirium.

Introduction

Case study: Janet's story

My name is Janet and I have been qualified as a nurse for one year. I normally work in the local burns unit, but we had only two patients that night and I found I had been allocated to work on an acute medical ward. I wasn't very familiar with the ward, but after a few hours I began to feel that I was comfortable with the layout and had assessed the patients I had been allocated. That was until midnight when I heard a scream coming from the female section followed by several shouts for help. I rushed down to see what was happening to find that a gentleman from the male section was attempting to get into bed with one of the female patients. The gentleman was pushing Joan (the female patient) out of bed to make room. I pulled her buzzer to call for assistance and tried to calm the situation down. The gentleman's name was Jack Porter (85 years), and at the time I knew nothing about him. I tried to reason with him and explained that he should go back to his bed where he would be more comfortable. He looked at me and nodded, and then walked over to another patient and tried to get into bed with her. I tried to talk to him again and gently held his elbow to steer him away. When I did this he resisted in an aggressive manner, pushing me and pinning me against the wall. The other staff again tried to reason with him, but he began shouting and pushing them away. Someone called for the on-call medical team to attend, and together we were able to calm Jack and persuade him to go back to bed. The medical team prescribed haloperidol and said they would perform a detailed assessment in the morning.

The female patients were terrified by this time and particularly frightened of the fact that it took three nurses and two medics to resolve the situation. No person came to physical harm that night, but the psychological distress felt by the female patients led to a disturbed and sleepless night for them. Jack was also clearly distressed and appeared to believe that we were going to harm him. After Jack had calmed and I had a chance to reflect, I realised that I was still shaking after the ordeal and that I needed to understand more about what had just happened so that I could manage such a situation better next time.

Janet's story is not uncommon and describes an example of a patient with acute confusion or delirium. According to NICE (2010a), in the UK the prevalence of delirium is 20–30% in medical wards and 10–50% in surgical wards. In ICU the incidence of delirium in ventilated patients is between 55% and 69% (Page, 2008). According to the National Clinical Guideline Centre (2010) patients who develop delirium have:

- a higher than average incidence of complications such as falls and pressure sores;
- a correspondingly increased length of stay in hospital;
- an increased incidence of dementia;
- an increased risk of mortality.

The importance of recognising, responding to and, where possible, preventing delirium cannot be overestimated, and in the remainder of the chapter we will explore how delirium can be assessed, diagnosed, prevented and managed.

What is acute confusion and how should it be described?

Acute confusional state, acute confusion and delirium are all terms used to describe an altered state of consciousness that is accompanied by a change in cognition or perception. The onset is acute, developing over one to two days and the course of the condition fluctuates according to time and other factors (American Psychiatric Association, 2000; NICE, 2010a, 2010b). The core features of delirium found in patients include:

- a reduced awareness and understanding of their immediate environment;
- an impaired ability to focus their attention, sustain and change their attention to something else;
- altered cognition, including: memory impairment, disorientation, paranoia, language or perceptual disturbances including hallucinations.

These disturbances develop over several days and tend to fluctuate during the course of the day. For example, acute confusion may only be manifested after dark and can be referred to as sundown syndrome (Beel-Bates and Rogers, 1990).

For some patients delirium will last a few days; for others it can continue for months, depending on the predisposing and precipitating factors listed in Table 8.2 on pages 154–5. The three subtypes of delirium described by NICE (2010a) are set out in Table 8.1.

What causes delirium?

Delirium appears to occur when a single factor or a combination of factors leads to a reversible organic mental syndrome. This means that in more than 90% of patients the underlying cause is physical and/or physiological, related to the impact of the disease and/or the impact of hospitalisation (Aldemir et al., 2001).

Delirium is triggered when the levels of neurotransmitters in the brain become altered (Borthwick et al., 2006). The main neurotransmitters and receptors that trigger delirium include:

- *dopamine*: helps to control the brain's reward and pleasure centres, regulate movement and emotional response;
- *acetylcholine*: plays a role in enhancing sensory perceptions when we wake up and in sustaining attention as well as regulating digestion and muscle movement;
- *serotonin*: plays a role in sleep, memory and learning, mood, behaviour and depression;
- *nicotinic and opioid receptors*: neuroreceptors that are associated with addiction;
- *bacterial infection* and endotoxins released as the bacteria breakdown can alter cell function in the brain.

Delirium subtype	Clinical signs	Patient examples
Hyperactive	Agitated and restless • Fidgeting. • Pulling at clothes, catheters or tubes. • Moving from side to side. • Shouting and calling out. Disorientated. • Doesn't know who or where they are. • May have difficulty following commands. Paranoia • Sees some members of staff as a threat. • Expresses fear and distress as the environment appears hostile. • May try to escape. Pain may be expressed as severe. Evidence of abnormal vital signs and imbalance in fluid and electrolytes.	Charlie Thomas (78 years) was admitted to a cardiac ward after feeling light-headed and dizzy. When he was admitted, his heart rate was 35/min and the ECG showed he had a bradycardia and complete heart block. A temporary pacing wire was inserted and his heart rate and blood pressure improved. Later that night the nurse noticed that his ECG trace had gone flat. She rushed to his bedside to find Charlie out of bed and looking for the exit. He had disconnected himself from the ECG leads but the pacing wire and equipment were still connected. He pushed past the nurse and made his way along the corridor towards the bus stop, wearing only pyjama bottoms. When the nurse caught up with him, he couldn't understand why he had to go with her because he needed to go home – they were expecting him. The nurse sat at the bus stop with Charlie for ten minutes before he agreed to come back to the ward and wait there.

Table 8.1: Subtypes of delirium with clinical examples

Continued

Delirium subtype	Clinical signs	Patient examples
Hypoactive	Disorientated • Doesn't know who or where they are. • May have difficulty following commands. Withdrawn • Lying quietly • Looking away and avoiding opportunities for human contact. • Evidence of abnormal vital signs and imbalance in fluid and electrolytes. This subtype is often difficult to diagnose and needs careful assessment from advanced assessment tools such as the Confusion Assessment Method for the ICU (CAM-ICU) (Ely et al., 2010).	Molly Adams (83 years) was quiet and withdrawn after her admission yesterday afternoon. She had been found by the postman lying in the hall after having fallen when trying to let the cat out. The door had got stuck open on the carpet so she had been lying in the cold for several hours. Molly had a fractured neck of femur and was waiting for surgery to stabilise the fracture. She didn't want to talk and when asked about her home arrangements she began to give information that was contradictory to what was in the nursing notes. When Molly was asked to roll on her side she didn't move or attempt to help with the procedure and she appeared not to understand simple commands. The nurse noted that this was very different from what she was like on admission when she was alert and keen to know who everyone was.
Mixed	The patient presents with a combination of hyper- and hypoactive signs often at different times in the day.	Chester Smith (90 years) was admitted to a surgical ward following an episode of acute abdominal pain; he was diagnosed with appendicitis and had emergency surgery that afternoon. In the post-operative period he appeared vague and withdrawn, and the staff thought that he had dementia. When his granddaughter visited, however, she said that normally he was as 'bright as a button' and that this was unusual behaviour for him. Later that night Chester began to get increasingly agitated, pulling at his urinary catheter and shouting for help. When the nurse tried to assess him, Chester began to shout even louder and pulled his urinary catheter out, throwing it on the floor.

Table 8.1: Continued

Some factors that trigger delirium are predisposing, in that some patients have increased risk of developing delirium before they have been admitted to hospital. This may be due to cognitive impairment, old age, pre-existing illness or functional impairment including vision or hearing loss. Delirium can also be caused by precipitating factors associated with the severity of the patient's illness, the use of certain drugs, electrolyte and chemical imbalance and sepsis. A full list of the predisposing and precipitating factors can be found in Table 8.2, which includes some clinical examples.

Why did Jack Porter develop delirium?

After the incident with Jack, Janet decided to read his notes and try to understand why he behaved the way he did. She found the following predisposing and precipitatory factors:

*   Predisposing.
    *   Age: Jack is 83 years old.
    *   He has been married to his wife for 62 years, and during that time they had never been separated for more than a few days. They are retired farmers.
    *   Jack has type II diabetes and hypertension for which he takes a beta blocker (slows the heart rate and reduces cardiac output).
    *   Jack had been admitted to hospital with a recent history of blackouts.
*   Precipitating.
    *   Jack has been in hospital for five days.
    *   His medication has been reviewed and reduced.
    *   He has been diagnosed with a urinary tract infection and prescribed antibiotics.
    *   His blood results from earlier today showed a raised sodium and potassium level, and an elevated creatinine level consistent with impaired renal function.
    *   When Jack settled, his respirations were 20/min, his pulse was 58/min and his blood pressure was 110/65mmHg (lower than normal for Jack); his temperature was 37.5°C and his blood sugar was 7.4mmol/l.
    *   Jack had only passed 500mls of urine in the last 18 hours.

Janet felt concerned for her patient and used the SBAR tool to ask the on-call medical team to review him that night instead of waiting until the morning. He was reviewed and commenced on an infusion of dextrose/saline to improve hydration and was catheterised in order to monitor his urine output. His medication for hypertension was reduced again due to his impaired renal function.

Activity 8.1   *Decision-making*

When you are next on placement in a hospital setting:

*   review the patients that you have been allocated for risk factors associated with developing delirium;
*   if you identify a patient who is at risk, collaborate with the health care team and discuss possible options for prevention as shown in Table 8.3;
*   continue to observe your patients to monitor any change in their condition that may increase the risk of them developing delirium.

As this activity is based on your own observation, there is no outline answer at the end of the chapter.

Predisposing factors	Clinical examples
Age	Any person, male or female who is 65 years or older, has an increased risk of developing delirium.
Existing cognitive impairment	Patients with existing dementia or depression have an increased risk of developing delirium.
Evidence of increasing severity of illness	A patient with bronchitis who develops an acute chest infection has an increased risk of developing delirium.
Existing physical impairment	Patients with visual and/or hearing impairments or with limited mobility can experience sensory deprivation in hospital, and this predisposes them to developing delirium.
Pre-existing alcohol/substance abuse	A person who may have abused drugs in the past but has not taken them for several years is still at risk of developing delirium as addiction can effect permanent changes on brain cells.

Precipitating factors	Clinical examples
Disease: • Respiratory disease and associated hypoxia (Chapters 2 and 3). • Cardiovascular disease. • Hypotension. • Severe infection. • Sepsis. • Head injury. • Acute admission for fractures and hip surgery. Physiological imbalance: • Imbalance of electrolytes particularly sodium and potassium.	• Hanna Mera (67 years) developed hyperactive delirium after her oxygen saturations fell to 87% as the result of an acute exacerbation of her chronic respiratory disease. • Harold Jones (70 years) developed delirium following a delayed diagnosis of myocardial infarction and hypotension. • Sarah Moon (65 years) developed delirium after developing sepsis from a wound infection. • Fred Holloway (78 years) fell and fractured his hip. He had to wait 48 hours after admission before he had surgery to stabilise the fracture. • Fred Holloway developed delirium post-operatively and he was found to have an imbalance in sodium and potassium, dehydration and an increase in his creatinine levels.

• Increased levels of creatinine, urea. • Anaemia. • Metabolic acidosis. • Dehydration. • Vitamin deficiency. • Blood glucose. Pharmacology: • Polymedication. • Drug withdrawal. • Drug side effects that cause an altered balance of the neurotransmitters acetylcholine and dopamine. • Failure to provide adequate pain relief. Use of physical and invasive therapy: • Physical restraint caused by equipment. • Indwelling catheters. • Immobilisation. • Lack of sleep. • Alien environment such as ICU.	• Mary Smith was admitted to hospital with cellulitis and sepsis. She was suffering from hypoxia and metabolic acidosis. She was disorientated and distressed. • Ryan Sheppard (20 years) was involved in a road traffic collision. He sustained multiple fractures. He was intubated and ventilated for 24 hours in the post-operative period, after which attempts were made to reduce his respiratory support. As he awoke he appeared to be hyper alert and tried to get out of bed. He was unable to respond to requests to stay in bed and became very agitated. Ryan was a regular user of illegal substances and that, together with his critical illness, had triggered delirium. • Barry Jones (54 years) had been a patient in ITU for 14 days, during which time he had been both physically restrained by catheters and tubes as well as chemically restrained by sedation to support respiratory function. He slept all day and was awake all night. At night he became very agitated and would regularly disconnect his ventilator tubing and attempt to get out of bed.

Table 8.2: Predisposing and precipitating factors for the development of delirium with clinical examples

How is delirium assessed and prevented?

When a patient is admitted to the ward or unit, part of their assessment on admission should include an assessment of the predisposing and precipitating risk factors for developing delirium.

As with all other elements of assessment, patients should be assessed using the 'Look: Listen: Feel: Measure' criteria. In this case it is very important to include information from the patient's friends and relatives in order to develop a picture of the patient as a person before they were admitted to hospital. Plan and organise the patient's care so that they see familiar faces among the carers, as this will provide continuity of care and continuity of assessment and monitoring. Assess for the core features of delirium (Table 8.1), and if any of these are present, your findings need to be validated by a more comprehensive clinical assessment such as the Confusion Assessment Method (CAM) (Ely et al., 2010; NICE 2010b). If a diagnosis of delirium is confirmed, the next step is to adopt a multidisciplinary approach to prevent further deterioration and treat any underlying precipitating factors. This process may be summarised as follows.

- Assess the patient and family using a holistic approach to care.
- Risk assess for predisposing factors for developing delirium.
- Promote continuity of care.
- Assess for features of delirium and, if present, validate with the use of an assessment tool (CAM).
- Risk assess daily for evidence of any changes in risk factors.
- Develop a multidisciplinary plan to risk assess and adopt preventative interventions.

Table 8.3 provides an example of a multidisciplinary plan for assessing and preventing delirium, using Jack Porter as an example.

Jack Porter remained in hospital for three weeks, and he remained in a state of delirium for a week before a gradual improvement was seen. After his discharge Jack was able to go home to his wife with support from community and social services. For patients in acute care, and particularly those patients who have undergone surgery, identifying the risk of delirium and preventing long-term problems for patients has become a priority (NICE, 2010a, 2010b). Your role as a nurse is to be vigilant in the holistic assessment of the patient and family in order to identify the potential for delirium and prevent it if possible.

The incidence of delirium among patients in ICU is up to 30% higher than found in acute medical and surgical wards. In the next section we will explore the relationship between the ICU environment and the development of delirium.

Case study: Paul Chapman

Paul Chapman (28 years) was on his way home from a night out when he was hit from behind by a hit-and-run driver. He was found by a passer-by who called the emergency services. Paul was taken to A&E where he was stabilised and transferred to the operating theatre. Paul's injuries included:

- *facial fractures;*
- *fractured ribs (3 and 4) on the left side and contusion on the right side of his chest;*
- *fractured pelvis;*
- *fractured right shaft of femur, tibia and fibula.*

In theatre Paul received the following.

- *External fixation of a fractured pelvis.*
- *Internal fixation and pinning of his right shaft of femur, tibia and fibula.*

Paul was transferred to ICU from theatre in an unconscious state, intubated and ventilated.

Factors on assessment	Preventative interventions	Preventative interventions for Jack Porter

Cognitive impairment Disorientation	• Reorientate the person by explaining:
	  • where they are
	  • who they are
	  • what your role is.
	• Provide:
	  • a clock
	  • a calendar
	  • appropriate signage
	• Provide cognitive stimulation:
	  • reminiscence
	• Encourage regular family visits
		• When Jack awoke the next morning we reminded him where he was and why.
		• We found his watch in the locker and put it on his wrist, checking it was the right time.
		• We explained what day it was and encouraged him to talk about his wife and family.
		• We contacted Jack's family to explain that he had become confused in the night and encouraged them to visit.

Hypoxia	• Assess for hypoxia and treat as necessary with oxygen, other medication, positioning and physiotherapy.	• Jack's oxygen saturations were 94% and we encouraged him to sit up and take regular deep breaths to help his breathing and circulation.
Dehydration Constipation	• Assess fluid balance and bowel activity daily • Encourage the person to take oral fluids; however, if necessary, supplement with subcutaneous or intravenous fluids	• Because of Jack's reduced urine output and elevated blood levels of sodium, potassium and creatinine, he was given an infusion of fluids to improve his fluid and electrolyte balance. • Jack had a history of cardiovascular disease so his respirations, pulse and fluid balance were monitored closely in case of fluid overload. • Jack's blood results were checked the next day to review the situation.
Imbalance in: electrolytes creatinine Metabolic acidosis	• Monitor blood levels of electrolytes, liver and renal function. • Assess for signs of metabolic acidosis (Chapter 3).	

Table 8.3: Clinical assessment factors and interventions to prevent delirium

Continued

Factors on assessment	Preventative interventions	Preventative interventions for Jack Porter
Infection	• Undertake daily infection and sepsis screening and escalate care as necessary (Chapter 7). • Implement infection control procedures. • Avoid invasive catheterisation unless necessary.	• The results from Jack's catheter specimen of urine directed a change in antibiotic therapy. • The presence of the urinary catheter was reviewed daily. • The catheter was removed three days later. • All infection control procedures were followed.
Multiple medications	• Review the person's medications and assess the risks of side effects and continued requirement for the drugs.	• Jack remained on a low dose of blood pressure medication and metformin for his diabetes.
Medications that alter the balance of neurotransmitters: • Anticholinergics: atropine, ipratropium bromide • Analgesics: morphine • Corticosteroids: hydrocortisone • Antihistamines: chlorphenamine • Cardiovascular agents: Dioxin, dopamine • Hypnotic drugs: diazepam	• Many of the drugs on this list will be vital for the patient's safety and well being. • It is important that the drugs are only given when necessary and reviewed daily.	• These were reviewed daily by checking blood glucose levels and vital signs.

Pain	• Assess for pain using a holistic approach and manage effectively.	• We continued to assess Jack for evidence of pain and discomfort.
Poor nutrition	• Undertake a nutritional assessment and assess factors that may be affecting adequate nutrition such as ill-fitting teeth.	• Jack's appetite had reduced since being diagnosed with a urinary tract infection. However, over the next few days he gradually improved.
Limited mobility	• Encourage patients who have had surgery to mobilise as soon as possible after surgery. • Encourage people to walk, with support if necessary, as often as possible during the day. • Encourage all patients to carry out active range of movement exercises every day.	• Jack was encouraged to walk around his bed and do a range of motion exercises during the day.
Sensory impairment	• Ensure hearing impairments are assessed and managed. • Ensure people have the appropriate glasses for reading and long-distance vision. • Provide regular stimulation for those patients who are physically isolated.	• We encouraged the family to bring in Jack's reading glasses as well as his regular spectacles so that he could read the paper.
Sleep disturbances	• Avoid undertaking medical and nursing procedures during sleep periods. • Reduce noise to a minimum.	• We kept Jack in the same section of the ward that he was used to and provided an environment to promote restful sleep.

Table 8.3: Continued

Activity 8.2   *Decision-making*

Using Table 8.2 as a guide, identify what information you would need to risk assess Paul Chapman for predisposing factors towards developing delirium.

You will find the answer later within the chapter.

In the next section you will find a summary of what happened to Paul in the first 36 hours following his accident.

Case study: Paul Chapman: the first 36 hours

When Paul was admitted to the accident and emergency unit he was suffering from:

- *hypoxia;*
- *hypovolaemic shock (Chapter 6);*
- *metabolic acidosis (Chapter 3).*

He was resuscitated with oxygen, respiratory support and fluid replacement, including a blood transfusion. Paul had been conscious at the scene, but his level of consciousness had deteriorated by the time he was admitted to hospital.

In ICU he was:

- *intubated with a tracheostomy tube to prevent destabilisation of his facial fractures;*
- *ventilated on bilevel pressure ventilation (Chapter 3).*

He had:

- *a central line;*
- *a peripheral infusion;*
- *an arterial line;*
- *ECG monitoring;*
- *a urinary catheter;*
- *a chest drain to drain a pneumothorax on his left side;*
- *medication for sedation and pain relief.*

Paul had several assessments of his haemoglobin, electrolyte function, renal and liver function, and any variation from the normal value was assessed and corrected. He continued to be sedated and ventilated, adhering to the ventilator bundle (Chapter 3).

Paul's family visited every day, and they agreed to divide the time between them so that there was someone there for him if he woke up or his condition changed.

When Paul was assessed for predisposing factors for the development of delirium, the nurse's initial assessment revealed that the only predisposing factor was that of his increasing severity of illness. This was reviewed, however, when Paul's mother confided in the nurse at the bedside that Paul had experimented with drugs as a teenager but had given them up eight years ago when he met his wife. This highlights the requirement to continually review your assessments – often not all the relevant information is available from the outset. This finding became significant when 48 hours later Paul was stable enough for the team to reduce his sedation and respiratory support.

Activity 8.3   *Decision-making*

Using Table 8.2 as a guide, assess Paul Chapman's risks for precipitating factors towards developing delirium.

An outline answer can be found at the end of the chapter.

Case study: Paul Chapman's sedation is reduced

As Paul started to wake up he became very agitated, and in spite of the use of reorientation and reassurance from Jenny, his nurse, Paul tried to pull out his peripheral and arterial line and ECG leads. Jenny continued to reassure him, explaining where he was and what had happened. She asked him if he had any pain, and Paul responded by beckoning to her to come closer. As Jenny leant forward Paul grabbed her round the waist and wouldn't let go. Jenny instinctively leant back and as she did so Paul came forward in the bed and was in danger of falling out. Jenny shouted for help, and with gentle reassurance from several members of staff Paul eventually let go and appeared to relax. A few minutes later, however, Paul was again trying to pull off anything that appeared to be attaching him to the bed. Jenny decided to invite Paul's sisters to the bedside in the hope that this would reassure him. She explained to his relatives why he was more awake and that he was quite agitated at times, but if he was able to settle, they would be able to reduce the sedation and respiratory support as the next step in his recovery. When Paul saw his sisters he held out his arms, and his elder sister Janice went forward to hold his hands. Paul, seeing her come closer, made a grab for her and pulled her onto the bed. We advised her to stay still and tried to persuade Paul to let her go. Paul resisted, and a team decision was made to recommence sedation and review the plan for weaning Paul from respiratory support. Paul's sister Janice was tearful and upset by what had happened, and Jenny tried to reassure her that this situation can occur in critically ill patients and that as Paul began to improve he would become less confused about what had happened.

Treating delirium

For some patients risk assessment and preventative interventions are not enough to prevent severe cases of hyperactive delirium. In the case study, Paul Chapman was suffering from severe symptoms of hyperactive delirium triggered by multiple predisposing and precipitatory factors. In cases such as Paul's, a plan of management would begin by dealing with the immediate problem of his distress. Paul was placing himself and others in danger by his actions, and the only option available was to recommence sedation with an infusion of midazolam in order to stabilise his condition and protect the safety of others. This can be described as a form of chemical restraint, which in Paul's case was justified in order to protect his safety in the short term (Bray et al., 2004).

When patients develop delirium a treatment plan should always begin with an assessment of the underlying causes and the provision of open and reassuring communication to both the patient and family (Borthwick et al., 2006; NICE 2010b). The causes of Paul's delirium were related to a history of drug abuse and factors related to his condition, such as fear and anxiety, physical restraint from his multiple therapeutic interventions such as the tracheostomy tube, ECG, infusions and urinary catheter, and the risk of physiological imbalance associated with his critical illness. The most effective method for managing Paul's delirium was to promote recovery and rehabilitation and the subsequent removal of trigger factors. According to Borthwick et al. (2006), patients with a history of drug abuse and who undergo sedation with benzodiazepines such as midazolam for seven days or more are very likely to experience delirium from their withdrawal. For Paul, a plan for recovery included a gradual reduction of sedation of several days and a daily review of his risk factors for developing delirium. Five days later Paul was awake and no longer requiring respiratory support. He was transferred to the orthopaedic ward where his rehabilitation continued. Paul continued to experience episodes of confusion for several months following his accident and, according to Arend and Christensen (2009), Paul may experience prolonged neuropsychological side effects that can extend beyond his physical recovery.

Key steps in treating delirium include:

* assess patient safety immediately;
* risk assess underlying causes;
* communicate with, reorientate and reassure the patient;
* consider involving family and friends;
* ensure stability and continuity of care using a team approach;
* if the patient is distressed, try verbal and non-verbal reassurance to calm the patient;
* if the patient's distress continues, consider the use of short-term medication such as haloperidol. This drug works by helping to correct the balance of dopamine and acetylcholine activity in the brain (Borthwick et al., 2006).

Chapter summary

Within this chapter we have considered the common causes of delirium (acute confusion) in patients placed in acute and critical care areas. We have explored ways in which patients can be risk assessed for developing delirium and how it may be prevented and treated. The key messages from this chapter to apply to your practice are the following.

* Patients who develop delirium have increased risk of morbidity and mortality.
* Daily risk assessment of patients for developing delirium can prevent its onset and should be considered a priority of care.
* Promoting good communication and continuity of care is an important factor in preventing delirium.
* If delirium cannot be prevented, then strategies and interventions used must be patient centred and enhance the safety of the patient and others.

Activities: brief outline answers

Activity 8.3: Decision-making (page 161)

Paul had the following precipitating factors.

- Disease:
    - damage to his lungs increasing the risk of hypoxia;
    - risk of hypotension associated with blood loss from his fractures;
    - emergency admission with multiple fractures.
- Physiological imbalance:
    - risk of anaemia;
    - risk of fluid and electrolyte imbalance associated with his injuries.
- Pharmacology:
    - prolonged period of anaesthesia and sedation
- Physical and invasive therapy:
    - intubation and ventilation;
    - a central line;
    - a peripheral infusion;
    - an arterial line;
    - ECG monitoring;
    - a urinary catheter;
    - immobilisation;
    - a chest drain to drain a pneumothorax on his left side;
    - alien environment;
    - disturbed sleep pattern.

Further reading

Arend, E and Christensen, M (2009) Delirium in the intensive care unit: a review. *Nursing in Critical Care*, 14(3): 145–54.

This paper provides a more in-depth discussion of the issues concerning patients with delirium in ICU.

Bray, K, Hill, K, Robson, W et al. (2004) British Association of Critical Care Nurses' position statement on the use of restraint in adult critical care units. *Nursing in Critical Care*, 9(5): 199–212.

This paper provides advice by the BACCN on the use of physical and chemical restraint for patients who become agitated and combative.

Useful websites

www.icudelirium.co.uk/

This website offers general information about the assessment, prevention and management of delirium and in particular a list of commonly used medications that can trigger delirium.

www.mc.vanderbilt.edu/icudelirium/assessment.html

This website has educational resources on how to assess patients using the confusion assessment method CAM-ICU. The site also provides links to videos that demonstrate the assessment in practice.

www.nice.org.uk/cg103

This website provides you with all NICE guidance documentation of assessing and treating delirium, including a guideline for patients and carers.

Chapter 9
The patient with altered consciousness

Jane James with Sandra Miles

NMC Standards for Pre-registration Nursing Education

This chapter will address the following competencies:

Domain 3: Nursing practice and decision-making

Generic competencies:

7. All nurses must be able to recognise and interpret signs of normal and deteriorating mental and physical health and respond promptly to maintain or improve the health and comfort of the service user, acting to keep them and others safe.

Field-specific competencies:

7.1. Adult nurses must recognise the early signs of illness in people of all ages. They must make accurate assessments and start appropriate and timely management of those who are acutely ill, at risk of clinical deterioration, or require emergency care.

NMC Essential Skills Clusters

This chapter will address the following ESCs:

Cluster: Care, compassion and communication

1. As partners in the care process, people can trust a newly registered graduate nurse to provide collaborative care based on the highest standards, knowledge and competence.

By entry to the register:

viii. Demonstrates clinical confidence through sound knowledge, skills and understanding relevant to field.

ix. Is self-aware and self-confident, knows own limitations and is able to take appropriate action.

Cluster: Organisational aspects of care

9. People can trust the newly registered graduate nurse to treat them as partners and work with them to make a holistic and systematic assessment of their needs; to develop a personalised plan that is based on mutual understanding and respect for their individual situation promoting health and well-being, minimising risk of harm and promoting their safety at all times.

continued . . .

By entry to the register:

xx. Acts autonomously and appropriately when faced with sudden deterioration in people's physical or psychological condition or emergency situations, abnormal vital signs, collapse, cardiac arrest, self-harm, extremely challenging behaviour, attempted suicide.

xxi. Measures documents and interprets vital signs and acts autonomously and appropriately on findings.

Chapter aims

By the end of this chapter, you should be able to:

- identify causes of impaired consciousness;
- describe the clinical features of altered consciousness in relation to trauma, toxicity, cerebro-vascular and neurological problems, and the clinical implications for the patient;
- undertake a neurological assessment;
- diagnose and differentiate between possible causes of patient deterioration and identify most appropriate interventions;
- relate the clinical examples in the chapter to your own practice.

Introduction

Case study: Unconsciousness

Julia, a student nurse, was walking through the park with her friend on a cold wintry morning when they found a young man lying on the path. Julia approached with caution while calling to him. As she got closer, she could see that his eyes were closed and he was clearly breathing. He was snoring loudly and his breath smelled of alcohol. Julia assessed his responsiveness using AVPU (alert, responsive to voice or pain, or unresponsive) and was unable to rouse him by speaking loudly to him, by shaking him gently or by pinching his trapezius muscle. While Julia continued her assessment, her friend used her mobile phone to call for an ambulance. In order to open his airway, Julia lifted the young man's chin and tilted his head back until he stopped snoring. She watched and listened to his breathing and counted his pulse rate before looking in his eyes and using verbal and painful stimulation to get him to respond. Starting at his head, Julia quickly looked and felt for visible injury on the parts of his body that were accessible. She found bruises and swelling on his head, face and abdomen, and his skin was cold to touch. Her friend found a wallet nearby that contained photographic identification of the young man and the name Mark Spencer on it.

There are many possible reasons why Mark was lying on the ground, and it was most important for Julia and her friend not to put themselves at risk. After excluding any danger, Julia recognised her professional obligation to help, knowing it was important to assess Mark's condition quickly using AVPU followed by ABCDE (airway, breathing, circulation, disability, exposure/environment/ everything else) (see Chapter 1) and to get help. She knew of several reasons for unresponsiveness, and that more detailed assessment would yield clues as to what had happened to Mark.

Julia's experience highlights the fact that patients with altered consciousness may not be able to give information to help with their assessment. Patients with altered conscious states are vulnerable and at risk of deterioration, and even death, from untreated causes as well as being unable to protect themselves from other harm. Mark's unconsciousness might not have been due to alcohol. Any additional findings that Julia noted on her assessment could be significant, and it was most important for Julia to keep Mark safe from further harm. She could do this by getting expert help, by ensuring his airway, breathing and circulation are protected (ABC) and by looking for any additional disabilities (D) and any other environmental factors (E).

Julia found a young man unconscious in the park. She had no way of knowing the circumstances of the situation. She knew that she must keep him safe, get help and assess the degree of unconsciousness as well as look for signs of the cause. What can we learn from this? There are several important messages in Julia's story.

- In emergency situations, always ensure that you do not put yourself or others in danger.
- Use a systematic approach to assess the situation and look for clues as to the causes.
- Be non-judgemental and continue your assessment to the end as there may be more than one problem.
- Organise the people around you and get professional help.
- You may not be able to do anything other than keep the patient safe in the short term, but this can reduce risk of long-term complications.

This chapter gives an overview of the possible causes of unconsciousness. It examines in detail the care of three patients suffering with altered consciousness related to the three main areas of head injury, stroke and seizure. It looks at the underlying physiology, social psychology and ethical implications of all three patients in the context of risk assessment and collaborative management and care.

The chapter begins with an explanation of unconsciousness, leading to an overview of the knowledge and skills required to recognise, assess, prioritise and manage care for patients with altered consciousness. Neurological assessment skills are explored based upon the requirements of the Glasgow Coma Scale. Confusion is seen in this chapter as an indication of altered consciousness, but is discussed in detail in Chapter 8.

What are the causes of unconsciousness?

Unconsciousness is a state of unrousable unresponsiveness where the victim is unaware of their surroundings and no purposeful response can be obtained (Martin, 2010). The brain requires a constant supply of oxygenated blood and glucose to function. Interruption of this supply will cause unconsciousness within a few seconds and permanent brain damage in ten minutes as the brain tissue becomes ischaemic. Other causes of unconsciousness can manifest more slowly as the severity of the problem progresses. Even with a gradual decline in consciousness, if the cause is left unattended, unconsciousness will eventually result and the likelihood of permanent disability increases with the period of unconsciousness (Woodward and Waterhouse, 2009). Causes can be classified into four broad groups as detailed in Table 9.1.

Activity 9.1	*Critical thinking*

Look again at the case study with Mark Spencer. What possible causes of Mark's unconsciousness can you identify from those shown in Table 9.1?

A brief outline answer is given at the end of the chapter.

General cause	Possible root cause	Clinical examples
Problems with oxygenation causing hypoxia	• Asphyxiation/drowning/asthmatic attack. • Carbon monoxide poisoning – inhalation of noxious gasses. • Trauma/injury to lungs/pneumothorax. • Chest infection – sputum retention. Infection – increases oxygen consumption.	1. Liz had a severe asthma attack and the bronchospasm restricted the flow of air through her airways – she was irritable and restless. 2. Bob's gas fire was faulty and he suffered carbon monoxide poisoning – he was unresponsive when found. 3. Peter sustained broken ribs when a tree fell on him, causing pneumothorax and precluding him from taking deep breaths – he couldn't remember his phone number. 4. Sally has pneumonia and secretions have consolidated the bases of both lungs – she was confused and disorientated.
Problems with cerebral circulation	• Occlusion of carotid artery by plaque, clot or compression. • Occlusion of vertebral arteries due to hyperextension of the head. • Rupture of cerebral vessels as in sub-arachnoid haemorrhage. • Hypotension/low cardiac output or slow heart rate. • Increased intracranial pressure caused by cerebral oedema, tumour, bleed, hydrocephalus causing reduced cerebral perfusion.	1. Audrey suffered a transient ischaemic attack – she was incoherent and her face was drooping on the left, but she is better now. 2. Bill collapsed in the library when he was looking up to get a book from the top shelf. He recovered almost immediately. 3. Catherine felt an explosion in her head like an elastic band snapping. She had a massive headache and is now responding only to voice. 4. Jennifer feels dizzy every time she stands up. Yesterday she fainted at work when she was rushing. 5. Andrew has a shunt for drainage of hydrocephalus. He is becoming increasingly drowsy, his eyes are half closed and he doesn't seem to be able to concentrate – the doctor thinks his shunt is blocked.

Table 9.1: Causes of diminished consciousness

General cause	Possible root cause	Clinical examples
Metabolic problems	• Overdose of drugs/alcohol. • Hypoglycaemia. • Electrolyte imbalance. • Sepsis.	1. Ian drank a bottle of whisky and now his friends can't wake him up. 2. Sharon is a diabetic. She is shopping with her friend and is being uncharacteristically aggressive to everyone and cannot be consoled. 3. Sheilagh has had copious diarrhoea. She complained of thirst and headaches, became restless and agitated and has just had a fit – her blood results show high sodium levels. 4. Henry was admitted with confusion and a urine infection. He is now hypotensive, tachycardic and responding only to voice.
Central nervous system problems	• Epilepsy – convulsions (post-ictal). • Injury or insult to brain tissue. • Meningitis or encephalitis.	1. Robin had his medication changed and has had violent fits. He is now very sleepy and responding only to painful stimuli. 2. Diane was hit by a car some weeks ago and sustained brain stem injury. She is now breathing spontaneously, yawns a lot and makes moaning sounds. She opens her eyes but doesn't look at you and she goes rigid when stimulated. 3. Ruby's lumbar puncture shows meningitis. She is photosensitive, has a terrible headache and is confused, irritable and just wants to sleep.

Table 9.1: Continued

Julia had no way of knowing whether Mark's unconsciousness was sudden or gradual, but to assess Mark effectively, she had to consider all possible causes of unconsciousness. She must also be mindful that combinations of different causes may be present – for example, a head injury as well as the influence of alcohol or drugs.

Recognising signs of deteriorating consciousness quickly, and understanding the possible underlying causes, allows early detection of physiological problems and early instigation of correct treatment and care. This can prevent the development of unconsciousness and further risk. Mark's most immediate risk was obstruction of his airway and respiratory arrest leading to cardiac arrest. Julia recognised this and acted immediately by performing the head-tilt, chin-lift manoeuvre. She then continued with a more detailed neurological assessment.

Assessing conscious level

The two aspects of consciousness generally considered in nursing neurological assessment are arousal, which indicates function of the reticular activating system (RAS) in the brain stem, and awareness or cognition, which indicates function of the cerebral hemispheres. Varying degrees of unconsciousness can occur depending upon the cause and extent of brain dysfunction. Julia used AVPU as a rapid initial assessment followed by the Glasgow Coma Scale (GCS) (NICE, 2007a). This more detailed assessment helped to establish Mark's degree of unconsciousness and which neurological responses were affected. The AVPU assessment findings can be loosely equated to ranges of the GCS score (see Table 9.2), indicating the urgency for more detailed neurological assessment.

The GCS is a widely used neurological assessment tool recommended by Jevon (2008) in assessing patients with altered consciousness. It measures three indicators of neurological function.

- Eye opening (E).
- Verbal response (V).
- Best motor response (M).

Scores are attributed to each indicator (Table 9.3) and should be considered separately, but may also be combined to give the overall coma score. The highest possible score is 15 and the lowest is three. Woodward and Waterhouse (2009) define coma as a GCS of eight or less. Because Mark did not respond to painful stimulus when Julia did the AVPU score, it suggested his GCS was dangerously low, indicating a state of coma.

In addition to noting GCS, it is important to assess pupil size, shape and reaction to light, and limb movements as well as temperature, pulse, respiratory rate, blood pressure and oxygen saturations. Together, these will give more accurate indications of your patient's neurological deficits and degree of risk.

AVPU score	Approximate GCS score
Alert	14–15
Responds to voice	9–13
Responds to pain	4–8
Unresponsive	3

Table 9.2: AVPU and equivalent GCS scores

Source: Cook (2006)

Indicator	Score	If the patient . . .	When you . . .	Because . . .
Eye opening	4	Opens eyes spontaneously.	Approach your patient or gently touch them if there is known hearing impairment	This demonstrates arousal or wakefulness which is dependent upon the reticular activating system (a dense network of neurons) within the brain stem being fully functional.
	3	Opens eyes to speech.	Say something loud enough to elicit a response (e.g his/her name). Or Touch your patient's hand, arm or shoulder and shake gently.	Trauma or increased intracranial pressure could impair neurone pathways within the reticular activating system requiring increased sensory stimulation to evoke eye opening. Speech is used, then touch and lastly pain.
	2	Opens eyes in response to pain.	Exert a painful peripheral stimulus by using the side of a pen or pencil to apply pressure to the side of the nail bed on the finger for a short time. Or Exert painful central stimulus by pinching the trapezius muscle.	A central painful stimulus may result in the patient grimacing, thus closing the eyes. An initial peripheral stimulus could avoid misleading results if there is no response to speech or touch. The side of the finger, rather than the actual nail bed, is used in order to minimize damage. It is important to elicit the best response, so central pain may be applied.
	1	Does not open eyes to stimuli.	Apply painful central stimulus (trapezius pinch). If eye opening is not possible due to orbital swelling, you need to note this and write 'C' against 'none' on the neurological observation chart	Intracranial pressure or neural damage due to trauma could be severely impairing the function of the reticular activating system.
Verbal response	5	Is orientated	Ask questions about the time, place and person, e.g. what the month or year is, where they are and who they are. Avoid questions requiring only yes/no answers. If the patient is expressively dysphasic,	The highest level of consciousness requires a person to be totally aware of their surroundings, being orientated to time, place and person. Questions requiring only yes/no answers are not conclusive as answers can be predicted.

		write 'D' instead. It is not essential to know the exact day and date due to the disorientating effect of prolonged hospital stays and hospital transfers.	It is important to be able to recognise and distinguish between receptive and expressive dysphasia as these can detract from accurate assessment for orientation. More detailed observation may be required.
4	Is confused	Ask the questions above and the patient cannot answer correctly but is able to converse.	Deterioration of consciousness begins with impaired ability to think clearly, repetition, impaired perception and responsiveness with reduced memory of current stimuli relating to time, place and person in that order.
3	Uses inappropriate words	Ask the questions above. Single-worded answers or the inability to make a sentence of words is classed as inappropriate words.	The cerebral hemispheres of the brain are most susceptible to damage and are responsible for verbal and analytical abilities, perception of language and performance of speech. Poor comprehension and impaired ability to express thoughts into words could indicate reduced cerebral function.
2	Makes incomprehensible sounds	Apply painful central stimulus (trapezius pinch). Noises such as moans or grunting sounds are classed as incomprehensible.	This is a sign of further deterioration of cerebral function extending to deeper structures of the brain. There is usually associated psychomotor impairment at this stage.
1	Makes no attempt at verbal response to stimuli.	Apply painful central stimulus (trapezius pinch). If no verbal response is possible due to an endotracheal tube or tracheostomy (without a speaking valve) write 'T' against 'none'.	Stupor and coma are indicated by little or no spontaneous activity and by being unrousable and unresponsive to external stimuli. These are signs of advanced brain failure. Intubated patients cannot speak although they may be conscious. They may attempt to mouth words, which are often very difficult to determine, so alternative scores may be misleading.

Continued

Table 9.3: Glasgow Coma Scale: how to score

Source: based on information from Porth (1998) and Woodward and Waterhouse (2009).

Indicator	Score	If the patient . . .	When you . . .	Because . . .
Best motor response	6	Obeys commands.	Ask the patient to move arm or leg or stick tongue out. Avoid asking patient to squeeze your hand. Apply a central painful stimulus (trapezius pinch) if there is no motor response to speech or touch. If there are varying responses from the different limbs you must note the best arm response and record the appropriate score for the response. Deficits in individual limbs will be recorded separately under 'limb movement'.	This indicates how well the brain is functioning as a whole by testing the areas of brain that precipitate motor responses to sensory stimuli. Following commands indicates the ability to process instructions. Grasping is a primitive reflex that may happen spontaneously, thus giving misleading scores. Central painful stimulus used as peripheral pain may evoke a spinal reflex action.
	5	Localises to central pain.		Purposeful or semi-purposeful movements are known as localising. Localising may be asymmetrical and when associated with clouding of consciousness as a result of the RAS being squeezed, can indicate increased intracranial pressure. This causes downward displacement of the cerebral hemispheres and structures of the upper brain to the level of the tentorium cerebelli, a transverse fold in the meninges that separates the structures of the upper and lower brain.
	4	Flexes limbs *normally* in response to pain.		The oculomotor nerve emerges to control pupillary constriction around the mid brain and can become trapped if the pressure continues to increase. It is at this point when changes in pupil reactions to light might begin. Flexion of limbs in response to pain is less well targeted to the stimulus than localisation, and indicates advancing brain dysfunction. Fluctuating respiratory function may be noticed at this point, identified by yawning or irregular breathing patterns.
	3	Flexes limbs *abnormally* in response to pain.		Abnormal flexion or decorticate rigidity (see Figure 9.1, p174) may indicate a lesion in the cerebral hemisphere or internal capsule where motor neurones originate.
	2	Extends limbs in response to pain.		Extension or decerebrate rigidity (see Figure 9.1) can be an indication of a lesion in the diencephalon, mid-brain or pons. It can also result from severe metabolic disorders, hypoxia or hypoglycaemia.
	1	Does not respond.		

Table 9.3: Continued

Activity 9.2   *Evidence-based practice and research*

Take some time to read the anatomy and physiology of the central nervous system. Make a note of the main structures of the brain and identify the parts that contribute to the neurological functions tested by the three indicators used in the Glasgow Coma Scale assessment in Table 9.3.

Because you will find this in your anatomy and physiology textbooks, there will be no answer provided for this activity. However, you may find Table 9.3 useful in linking the pathophysiology to your practice.

Case study

When Julia assessed the three indicators of Mark's GCS, he did not open his eyes to central painful stimulus, nor did he make any vocal sounds. Julia noticed some flexion in response to trapezius pinch when Mark seemed to move his left arm upwards towards her hand. Checking a second time, she could also see that his left knee rose slightly. She considered this to be localising to pain, even though it was weak and only on one side of his body, thus scoring E1, V1, M5 (see Table 9.3). This gave a total score of 7 out of 15, confirming that Mark's conscious level was dangerously low and he was at risk of stopping breathing.

Julia had noted bruising and swelling of Mark's face, but was still able to lift his eyelids to look at the size and shape of his pupils. She opened both Mark's eyes at the same time in order to compare the pupil size and shape. Both were round, although the left pupil looked slightly larger than the right. Julia did not have a torch with her, so used her friend's mobile phone to shine a light directly at each pupil in turn. She moved the light across Mark's left eye, from the outer aspect to rest over the pupil, then back again and repeated this on the right side to check the right pupil. Noting each pupil response, Julia could see that the left pupil was slower to constrict than the right pupil, which moved so quickly that she could only really see it dilating when she took the light away. Julia made a point of repeating the observation, looking at the non-stimulated pupil, and noted that the right pupil still constricted quickly when light was shone into the left eye, but the left pupil remained sluggish in response when light was shone into the right eye.

Activity 9.3   *Evidence-based practice and research*

Take a torch with a bright white light and narrow beam, and ask a friend to allow you to shine it in their eyes, using the same technique as Julia.

1. Note what happens.
2. What are the difficulties in this technique of pupil assessment?
3. Look at Table 9.3. What might be happening to Mark to elicit the pupil response Julia noted? What might happen next?

An explanation of what you might notice and the answers to the questions can be found at the end of this chapter.

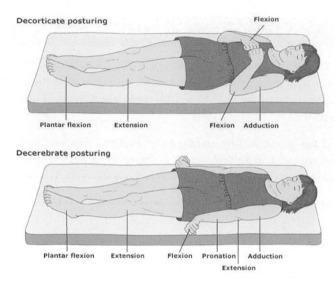

Figure 9.1: Decorticate and decerebrate posturing are examples of 'abnormal posturing'. They are involuntary flexion or extension of the arms and legs, indicating severe brain injury. They occur when one set of muscles becomes incapacitated while the opposing set is not, and an external stimulus such as pain causes the working set of muscles to contract. These types of posturing are indicators of the amount of damage that has occurred to the brain, and are used to measure the severity of a coma with the Glasgow Coma Scale.

Julia informed the paramedics of her findings on assessing Mark. They quickly undertook a further ABCDE assessment including GCS and secured Mark's airway with an endotracheal tube (see Chapter 3). This would allow them to administer oxygen and assist with his respirations should his consciousness deteriorate further, affecting the central areas of the brain that control the vital functions. Julia had kept Mark safe until professional help arrived.

In the A&E Department Mark's level of consciousness was reassessed according to the guidelines (NICE, 2007a). Blood tests and radiological investigations enabled the medical and nursing team to eliminate many of the causes of unconsciousness that you may have identified earlier. A computerised tomography (CT) scan should be performed immediately on patients with GCS less than 13, with results available within one hour (NICE, 2007b). It later emerged that Mark had been assaulted and kicked repeatedly in the head after leaving the pub where he had been for a drink with his friend the previous evening to celebrate his twenty-third birthday.

Even though there was no evidence of intracranial haematoma or skull fracture on the CT scan, Mark had suffered head trauma causing obvious external bruising and swelling, and his neurological assessment suggested changes to the cerebral hemispheres and oculomotor nerve that could be due to intracranial bruising and cerebral oedema.

What are the nursing priorities of the unconscious patient?

Case study: Head injury

David is a third-year student nurse on critical care placement in the intensive care unit. Penny, his mentor, agreed that he should look after a newly admitted patient in order to focus on priorities of care. They prepare a bed area for Mark, who was in A&E, having suffered a closed head injury following assault. He was to be sedated, ventilated and closely monitored for 24 hours. While Mark is being prepared for transfer, Penny asks David what would be the nursing priorities in caring for Mark.

David was aware that he and Penny would need to work collaboratively with the medical team to reduce the risk of death or long-term brain damage for Mark. Any initial damage to Mark's brain (primary damage) was irreversible, but the main objective was to prevent further (secondary) damage, as rising intracranial pressure (ICP) was the biggest threat to Mark.

A quick ABCDE assessment and response (see Chapter 1) would address any immediate dangers, but David really needed to know which aspects of care could affect Mark's ICP. He was unsure how to prevent further increase and how best to aid reduction of ICP. Penny points out some important specific nursing considerations to help with reducing the risk of secondary damage. These are identified in Table 9.4.

How can secondary brain injury be prevented?

Preventing secondary brain damage depends upon the quality and quantity of circulation to the brain. For Mark, this means having adequate oxygenation and blood pressure, and maintenance of normal ABGs and blood glucose levels. Increases in ICP result from cerebral oedema, infection, haematoma, tumour or hydrocephalus taking up space within the skull (Porth, 1998). Because the skull is rigid, the contents become squeezed and the intracranial pressure rises. Mark's raised ICP was due to cerebral oedema, which can subside naturally as healing processes take place. Sometimes intravenous infusion of hypertonic sodium chloride solution may be prescribed (Helmy et al., 2007). This uses osmosis to draw the fluid (with lower concentration) from the swollen brain tissue into the higher concentration fluid of the cerebral circulation to be returned to the central circulation, then excreted by the kidneys. In both cases the injured tissue needs to have a good blood supply for the swelling to reduce.

Intracranial pressure and arterial blood pressure work in opposition, so cerebral perfusion depends on the blood pressure being strong enough to counteract ICP. Thus, Mark's mean arterial blood pressure (MAP) must be high enough to counteract any rise in ICP. If Mark's MAP dropped too low, cerebral circulation would be compromised and his brain tissue would be poorly perfused, and poor perfusion can lead to further swelling, thus compounding the problem.

Problem	Intervention	Rationale
1. Cerebral oedema may increase during first 24–48 hours, causing ICP to rise further.	Keep sedated and minimise stimulation.	Prevents coughing, sneezing and straining which temporarily increase ICP.
	Nurse in a 15–30° head-up tilt.	To optimise cerebral venous drainage.
	Keep head in neutral alignment with body. Ensure ET tube ties are not tight around neck.	Avoids obstructing jugular veins which would prevent cerebral venous drainage.
	Avoid hip flexion.	Prevents raised intra-abdominal pressure leading to raised intra-thoracic pressure which in turn impedes cerebral venous drainage.
2. Inadequate oxygen delivery to the brain tissues will cause further cerebral damage and exacerbate oedema.	Care of ET tube. Perform endotracheal suction to remove secretions if needed.	Ensures airway remains patent and optimises gaseous exchange.
	Titrate inspired oxygen and ventilator settings against ABG and SaO_2 results to keep PaO_2 normal.	Optimises ventilation and avoids increased blood flow to the brain which takes up space and increase ICP.
	Keep sedated – monitor sedation score.	Reduces cerebral oxygen demand.
	Avoid infection – use aseptic techniques, monitor body temperature, and aim to keep it normal.	Raised body temperature increases O_2 demand and CO_2 production, thus increasing cerebral oxygen use. Patients with head injury are susceptible to chest infection, which can lead to sepsis. High ICP can squeeze the hypothalamus, causing temperature regulation to be lost.
3. Inadequate cerebral perfusion pressure (CPP) will compromise oxygen delivery to the brain, exacerbating cerebral oedema. Good perfusion is needed to help to reduce the cerebral oedema.	Monitor heart rate.	Changes in heart rate can indicate early B/P compensating mechanisms, increasing ICP or inadequate sedation, which may need to be acted upon. Cardiac dysrhythmias need correcting. They reduce efficiency of the heart causing hypotension.
	Monitor fluid input and output – replace fluids to prevent hypotension.	Ensures adequate circulating volume. Gives early identification of excessive diuresis (diabetes insipidus) resulting from pituitary gland being squeezed. Gives indication of renal function.
	Keep MAP <70mmHg and CPP <60mmHg. Titrate prescribed inotropic drugs to correct hypotension.	MAP counteracts rise in ICP to allow adequate cerebral perfusion pressure (CPP = MAP-ICP).
	Keep $PaCO_2$ on low side of normal.	Higher CO_2 levels cause vasodilation. This takes up space and increases ICP. Increased ICP reduces CPP.
	Use correct patient positioning and care of ET tube ties.	Avoids cerebral venous drainage, thus reducing cerebral vascular congestion.
4. Head injury can cause hyperglycaemia and increase metabolism.	Monitor and correct glucose levels as per policy.	Reduces mortality.
	Commence enteral feeding as soon as possible	Prevents catabolism (breakdown of complex substances to produce energy) which creates more CO_2.

Table 9.4: Priorities of care to prevent secondary damage in head injury

Imagine you are Mark's nurse in the A&E department. Using the SBAR communication tool (see page 20), make a note of the content and sequence of your handover to David and Penny in ICU.

A plan of Mark's handover can be found at the end of this chapter.

Case study

David and Penny prioritised Mark's care for the next 24 hours. Mark remained stable but his repeat CT scan showed evidence of cerebral oedema. It was agreed that he should be kept sedated and ventilated for a further 24 hours to allow this to settle down. When Mark's sedation was reduced, he was restless and agitated, requiring re-sedating. One day later, Mark became septic secondary to pneumonia. On day seven Mark's sedation was stopped and he was extubated successfully. He was not agitated, but his GCS remained low at 9/15 (E3, V2, M4) indicating residual brain damage. Mark's recovery from this point was very uncertain, and it was impossible to know whether the brain damage resulted from primary or secondary injury.

Being alert to subtle changes in patient behaviour

Scenario: Stroke

Imagine you are working on the rehabilitation ward and looking after Mrs Pam Green who suffered a haemorrhagic stroke ten days ago. This morning when you woke her she resisted getting out of bed and did not appear to be making her usual effort with her exercises. Communication can be difficult because of her expressive dysphasia, but today she did not appear to want to cooperate and she was yawning, so you left her in bed. You return two hours later to find Pam slumped in her bed. On assessment of her GCS, she scores 5 (E1, V1, M3) and her pupils are fixed and dilated. There is no response to light.

Consider Mrs Green's scenario and answer the following questions.

- What signs of altered consciousness were missed?
- What could these signs have indicated?
- What could have been done?
- Why do you think Pam did not get the required attention?

Answers to these questions can be found at the end of this chapter.

Mrs Green's deterioration appeared to be a sudden event, but clues were evident some time before she became unresponsive. You need to make objective assessments despite communication difficulties and avoid any preconceptions. You will come across situations similar to Mrs Green's in all spheres of nursing. It is important to be aware of the subtle changes in patient behaviour as these are the earliest indicators of altered consciousness. If you are alert to these changes, then early intervention may prevent deterioration in most cases.

Because Mrs Green had previously suffered a stroke and had some residual neurological deficits, continued assessment would not only identify any deterioration but could also be used to measure progress. Limb assessment may be specifically useful in this instance.

Limb assessment

Limb assessment usually forms part of the overall neurological assessment with the GCS, pupil responses and vital signs. Changes in limb movements can help to pinpoint more specifically the area and degree of brain injury, although it is important to eliminate any pre-existing conditions that may affect limb movement, such as previous stroke or injury (Woodward and Waterhouse, 2009). Ideally, the patient should be able to obey commands, so despite expressive dysphasia, Pam should have been able to respond. Some patients with receptive dysphasia may benefit from a demonstration of what is expected of them.

It is important to compare left side with right side of arms and then legs, rather than assess each limb independently, although results for each limb should be recorded separately. Pam could have been asked to lift her limbs against gravity or slight resistance. This is more useful than asking her to squeeze your hands as grasping is a primitive reflex and may give misleading results. Deviation from previous recorded findings is most significant and this may well have been revealing in Pam's scenario.

Spontaneous or involuntary movement should be recorded, as well as limb strength, which is classified as:

* normal – usual power and strength;
* mild weakness – inability to fully lift limbs or difficulty in moving against resistance;
* severe weakness – unable to lift limbs but can move them laterally.

Patients who are unable to obey commands can be assessed for limb movement in response to pain as in the 'best motor response' section of the GCS. Any difference between responses in left and right must be noted in the limb movement assessment.

Pam's condition was deteriorating when she seemed to be resisting care. A thorough GCS, including limb assessment, would have revealed that she opened her eyes to voice (E1), made incomprehensible sounds or inappropriate words (V2 or 3) and localised to pain (M5), but that her best motor response was weaker than her last limb assessment had shown. With this information, medical attention could have been summoned much earlier. Unfortunately, it is likely that Pam suffered another intracerebral bleed, and prognosis in this instance is extremely poor.

Seizure: what action is needed?

Seizures are transient episodes of neurological deficit and take many different forms depending upon their origin and cause. They are often associated with epilepsy, but can be triggered by drugs, alcohol, metabolic disorders, pre-eclampsia, head injury or cerebral hypoxia and pyrexia in children (Woodward and Waterhouse, 2009). Abnormal electrical activity can start in one part of the brain and spread, sometimes involving localised areas and sometimes affecting the whole cerebral cortex. Various symptoms result, depending upon the area and location of brain involvement.

Case study: Seizure

Student nurse Claire was returning to the ward from an errand when she met a young lady in the ward entrance. She seemed to be walking aimlessly, but on approach Claire established that she was visiting her mother, Mrs Watkins, who was a patient on the ward. Claire directed her to the correct bed, but saw her stop. She was fiddling with her hands, then collapsed on to the floor. Her arms were jerking and she was making choking sounds. Claire shouted for help and cleared the area of obstacles. She was unsure of what to do next and was relieved when the ward sister appeared.

This young lady was showing early signs of onset of seizure when Claire met her. The subtle behaviour that Claire noticed is significant and will be useful for Miss Watkins and her family members to recognise in future. The most important and immediate concern is to keep her safe for the duration of the seizure, using the ABCDE approach and to protect her from injury.

It is not recommended, or safe, to open the mouth of someone having a seizure to insert an oropharyngeal airway because of jaw clenching, and stimulation may further exacerbate the seizure. It is usual to allow short seizures to run their course, observing closely, and to intervene once the seizure stops (Woodward and Waterhouse, 2009). It is not advisable to restrain the victim. If seizures are continuous, prescribed emergency medication such as diazepam should be administered through an accessible route with quick absorption.

Activity 9.6   *Evidence-based practice and research*

Visit the International League Against Epilepsy website at www.ilae.org to find out more about the classification of seizures, current research and recommendations.

As this is your own research, there is no answer to this activity at the end of the chapter.

Case study: Seizure (continued)

Sister removed the scarf from around the neck of Miss Watkins and advised Claire to cushion her head with a pillow, and to make a note of the duration of the seizure and all the different components, such as noises, movements and progression, colour and injuries. The staff nurse arrived with emergency equipment and positioned herself at Miss Watkins's head, ready to protect her airway and support her breathing. Once Miss Watkins seemed to relax (after 75 seconds), Sister asked Claire to help her put Miss Watkins into recovery position. The staff nurse protected the airway using a head tilt and chin lift, and had oxygen and a face mask ready. The nursing team carried out a full set of observations, including temperature, pulse, respirations, blood pressure, oxygen saturations and neurological assessment. Miss Watkins began to respond after a further two minutes and was helped on to a bed to recover.

Sister found out from Mrs Watkins that her daughter suffered with epilepsy, and had recently had her medication regime reviewed.

Claire's experience could have happened outside the hospital where no emergency equipment is available. However, despite the help from experienced health care professionals, we can see that the initial actions required only common sense. Claire acted appropriately by:

- noting symptoms leading up to the seizure;
- calling for help;
- preparing a safe environment;
- staying with the patient;
- being prepared to intervene with the ABCDE approach afterwards.

The duration of seizures is often surprisingly short, so it is important to note components and timings of all the phases. The patient may not remember events, so information is useful for them and their families for future management and care. It is important to reassure the patient and to be able to provide accurate and reliable information regarding the cause of their seizures and their likely course. The nurse has a role in patient education and health promotion, as well as recognising signs of impending and actual problems.

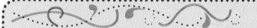

Chapter summary

This chapter highlights the nursing responsibilities of rapid and accurate neurological assessment and subsequent prioritisation of care for patients with altered consciousness and at risk of deterioration. Nurses can come across patients with altered consciousness in all clinical settings, and early intervention and prioritisation of care can reduce complications. Outcomes are not always good, but increased understanding of neurological problems will enable you to make evidence-based clinical judgements.

Activities: brief outline answers

Activity 9.1: Critical thinking (page 166)

Several of the causes identified in Table 9.1 could apply to Mark: alcohol intoxication; drug overdose; head injury; hypoglycaemia; hypotensive episode such as fainting; hypoxia; infection such as meningitis or encephalitis; post-ictal (post-fit); spontaneous intracranial bleed such as subarachnoid haemorrhage.

Activity 9.3: Evidence-based practice and research (pages 173–4)

1. Normally, when a bright narrow beam of light is shone into one eye and held there, the pupil of that eye constricts briskly to a pin-point size of about 1mm. The pupil dilates again, usually back to its original size, when the light is removed. To avoid misleading results in pupil size difference, it is important to check equality of pupil sizes prior to subjecting them to light stimulus. Normally, both pupils respond when light is shone in only one of them – this is the consensual response that helps to test the optic nerve.
2. Difficulties with this technique.
- You may find some healthy people have unequal pupils ordinarily.
  - With brown eyes it is sometimes difficult to determine the margin of the pupil from the iris, so the motor response may need to be noted from the dilation of the pupil on removing the light rather than looking for constriction on applying the light stimulus.
  - The brightness of light in the room, and the width and strength of the light beam affects starting pupil size and may hinder response.
  - Moving the light stimulus across the bridge of the patient's nose can hinder response, so it is better to introduce the light from the outer aspect of the eye.

- Patients who are photosensitive will find this very uncomfortable and may resist the assessment. Likewise, orbital oedema that precludes eye opening hinders assessment in the very patients who may need to be monitored.

3. Mark's direct pupil responses indicated that his optic and oculomotor cranial nerves were functioning. The fact that his left pupil was slow to constrict suggests that either the left optic nerve had impaired sensitivity to light, or that the conduction pathway of the left oculomotor nerve was impeded. The brisk consensual response of the right pupil when light was shone into the left eye demonstrates that the left optic nerve was sensing the light. These findings give strong clues as to the extent of intracranial pressure increase (see Table 9.3) and suggest that Mark's left oculomotor nerve was getting squeezed, and the intracranial pressure was such that the cerebral hemispheres were being pushed down towards the tentorium cerebelli. If the pressure continued to rise, the next sign would be a change in left pupil shape to oval, then a fixed and dilated left pupil, accompanied by reduced motor responses to painful stimuli and haemodynamic changes as the mid-brain and brain stem start to get squeezed. This is a dangerous situation for Mark.

Activity 9.4: Communication (page 177)

Introduce self and department.

Patient's name: Mark Spencer, 23-year-old male.

Situation

- Unconscious closed head injury.
- Intubated and ventilated.
- Bruising and swelling to head, face and abdomen.
- No other injuries.

Background

- Give home situation if known.
- Went out for a drink last night.
- Assaulted – kicked repeatedly in the head.
- Found unconscious in park this am – give original GCS – and has been unconscious since.
- No significant past medical history.
- Usually fit and well.
- Takes no medication.

Assessment

- Airway – intubated by paramedics at the scene.
- Breathing – spontaneously on admission, now sedated and ventilated. Give breathing rate, % oxygen delivered and oxygen saturations readings.
- Circulation – give heart rate, blood pressure, temperature measured and peripheral temperature to touch.
- Disability – give latest GCS score and pupil assessment, blood glucose result, CT scan and X-ray results. Summarise blood results and give any significant deviations from normal. Give information relating to medication and fluid administered and diuretic response to hypertonic saline if given.
- Exposure – if not already mentioned, give urine output and state if catheterised. Indicate other injuries and how they have been treated.

Response

Outline proposed plan

- Keep sedated and ventilated for next 24 hours.
- Repeat CT scan tomorrow to check for cerebral oedema.
- Repeat ABGs one hour after transfer.
- Keep PaO_2 normal and $PaCO_2$ on low side of normal.
- Give any information regarding family, police and property.
- Agree a time for transfer.

Activity 9.5: Critical thinking (page 177)

First of all, Mrs Green may not have been asleep, but she opened her eyes to vocal stimulation. Resisting getting out of bed and lack of effort and cooperation may not have been stubbornness but due to reduced awareness and cognition. Early signs of deterioration in consciousness include decreased concentration, agitation, dullness and lethargy (Porth, 1998). These fit with Pam's change in behaviour, but because of her usual expressive dysphasia, her falling GCS went unnoticed. Depending upon the degree of Pam's expressive dysphasia, it may be difficult to ascertain confusion and inappropriate words from incomprehensible sounds. Yawning is an early respiratory indicator of rising intracranial pressure (Porth, 1998).

Had Pam's GCS been thoroughly assessed, it should have been possible to note that she could not obey commands and that she was losing control of motor function. Assessment of vital signs, limb movement and pupil reactions may have helped to conclude findings.

It is not clear whether the course of Pam's deterioration could have been halted.

It is not safe to assume that recovering patients are safe from deterioration.

Further reading

Edwards, M and Griffiths, P (2011) *Emergency nursing made incredibly easy*. London: Lippincott Williams and Wilkins.

This book gives easy to understand explanations of emergency care and includes a specific chapter dedicated to neurological problems.

Geraghty, M (2005) Nursing the unconscious patient. *Nursing Standard*, 20(1): 54–56.

This article gives comprehensive coverage of the nursing management of unconscious patients, taking into account all activities of living based on lifelike scenarios.

Goulden, I (2011) Traumatic brain injury, in Clarke, D and Ketchell, A (eds) *Nursing the acutely ill adult: priorities in assessment and management*. Basingstoke: Palgrave Macmillan.

This chapter deals with traumatic brain injury, considering medical and surgical interventions in a clearly laid out format.

NICE (2007) *Head injury: triage, assessment, investigation and early management of head injury in infants, children and adults*. London: National Institute for Health and Clinical Excellence.

This gives comprehensive guidance on care of patients with head injury. Nurses involved in caring for acutely ill patients should have this information.

Useful websites

www.ilae.org/

The International League Against Epilepsy website presents a wealth of information about epilepsy. The different classifications and manifestations are explained. There are presentations, research papers and practice guidelines.

www.stroke.org.uk/

The Stroke Association website gives information for patients and professionals about the different stages of stroke. There are links to research articles as well as information and advice that you can pass on to your patients.

Chapter 10
The patient with physiological trauma

Catherine Williams with Susan Salerno

NMC Standards for Pre-registration Nursing Education

This chapter will address the following competencies:

Domain 3: Nursing practice and decision-making

3.1. Adult nurses must safely use a range of diagnostic skills, employing appropriate technology, to assess the needs of service users.

Domain 4: Leadership, management and team working

3. All nurses must be able to identify priorities, and manage time and resources effectively to ensure the quality of care is maintained or enhanced.

NMC Essential Skills Clusters

This chapter will address the following ESCs:

Cluster: Care, compassion and communication

1. As partners in the care process, people can trust a newly registered graduate nurse to provide collaborative care based on the highest standards, knowledge and competence.

Cluster: Organisational aspects of care

9. People can trust the newly registered graduate nurse to treat them as partners and work with them to make a holistic and systematic assessment of their needs; to develop a personalised plan that is based on mutual understanding and respect for their individual situation promoting health and well-being, minimising risk of harm and promoting their safety at all times.

16. People can trust the newly registered graduate nurse to safely lead, co-ordinate and manage care.

17. People can trust the newly registered graduate nurse to work safely under pressure and maintain the safety of service users at all times.

18. People can trust a newly registered graduate nurse to enhance the safety of service users and identify and actively manage risk and uncertainty in relation to people, the environment, self and others.

Chapter aims

By the end of this chapter, you should be able to:

- interpret the mechanisms of injury to form individualised patient care;
- demonstrate the systematic approach to physiological trauma care;
- describe the primary and secondary survey;
- list the indications for intravenous fluid replacement therapy;
- reflect on clinical examples illustrated in the chapter and apply this to your own clinical situation.

This chapter introduces you to the physical and psychological impact of trauma and about how to help patients and their families in their own processes of healing, recovery and restoration.

Case study

Mrs Doris Daniels, aged 74, is admitted to A&E after tripping over a raised paving slab while running for a bus. Lily, a student nurse, is working with her mentor, who is triaging patients in A&E. It is the first day of Lily's placement. On admission Mrs Daniels is carefully holding her left wrist and is able to give her own account of the accident, although she speaks slowly and deliberately as though she is trying to speak with loose dentures. She has an abrasive graze to her swollen nose and chin and a runny nose. Mrs Daniels appears embarrassed by her facial injuries and focuses on her wrist injury.

*Lily did not carry out an accurate primary assessment, GCS and history but focused upon the secondary survey assessment of Mrs Daniels. Lily assumes that Mrs Daniels' wrist probably has a **Colles fracture** because of the classic dinner fork deformity presentation. An X-ray will be needed to confirm this with subsequent reduction of the fracture.*

*However, Lily's mentor is a very experienced A&E nurse and she prioritises Mrs Daniels more urgently. After completing an accurate primary and secondary survey she believes that Mrs Daniels may have sustained maxillofacial injuries based on the abnormal facial mobility and may have a leak of **cerebrospinal fluid** (CSF) from her nose. CSF is clear and has a high sugar (clinistix) and low protein content (electrophoresis) compared to nasal or lacrimal fluid. If CSF is leaking due to a facial injury, the patient may complain of a persistent salty taste in the mouth. Neurological observations are commenced on Mrs Daniels and she is admitted to the resuscitation bay for urgent medical attention. If left untreated, the type of injuries that cause CSF leaks can represent a life-threatening situation and could lead to meningitis, brain infection, stroke and death. Maxillofacial trauma must be given the same priority as other head injuries.*

There are important messages to learn from Lily's story.

- Always be alert to changes in your patient's clinical condition, no matter how small. Any patient who has sustained an injury to the face or jaws should be suspected of having an actual head injury.

- The ABCDE order of treatment reflects the importance of the differing things that can go wrong, and the primary survey must be completed before moving on to address the obvious injuries. Poor tongue support in **mandibular** fractures can cause airway obstruction.
- Errors are often made in the early management of the trauma patient so a systematic approach is required in order to identify and treat the immediately life-threatening and potentially life-threatening conditions before the limb threatening ones.
- Timing is of the essence: your patient will continue to deteriorate if prompt action is not taken.

What do we mean by physiological trauma?

This chapter provides an overview of the general causes and treatments of physiological trauma, and examines in detail the care of a patient with physiological trauma and the metabolic response to trauma. The chapter proceeds with an overview of the knowledge and skills required to assess, differentiate and manage the care of a patient who sustains any form of physiological trauma. The underlying physiology and implications of the patient's care will be discussed in the context of diagnostic tests, treatments and collaborative management of care and highlighted through the chapter. The assessment and management of patients with shock is touched upon in this chapter; for a detailed assessment of **cardiogenic** and **distributive shock** (including sepsis and **septic shock**), please refer to Chapters 4, 6 and 7.

Trauma care starts at the point of injury and continues through to the end of rehabilitation to ensure the best possible outcome; in any trauma an organisational approach is essential.

What is trauma?

Eckes-Roper (cited in Saunderson-Cohen, 2003) defines trauma as a blunt or penetrating force to the body resulting in actual injury.

Irrespective of the cause of trauma, the medical team must make a systematic assessment in order to ensure that the most important injuries are prioritised. Courses such as the Advanced Trauma Life Support (ATLS) provide a means of assessing patients that is widely accepted worldwide as a framework of rapid assessment for trauma. Broadly speaking, this comprises a **primary survey** and a **secondary survey** of the patient to ensure that less obvious serious injuries are not missed while health care staff deal with more visually apparent patient problems. It is easy to become distracted by obvious injuries when there may be more immediately life-threatening injuries.

Types of trauma to the body can be classified as blunt or penetrating.

- Blunt trauma – can be caused by falls or seatbelt injuries but leaves the body surface intact.
- Penetrating trauma – can be caused by stab injuries and the body surface is damaged.

(Bersten and Soni, 2003)

A systematic approach to trauma management is a relatively recent (1970s) concept, and trauma care has been much improved with systematic approaches that enable effective treatment. Prior to this, survival of major trauma was less likely than it is today.

Case study

Danny, a seven-year-old boy was a front-seat passenger in his uncle's car. He was not in a car seat, and he was not wearing a seatbelt. As they drove along the road at around 30mph, Danny stood up and turned around to wave to the people in the car behind. At that point, his uncle braked heavily and swerved to avoid a car that had pulled out from a junction without looking. While the impact was not particularly serious, Danny was catapulted into the dashboard and had an obvious ankle deformity requiring a visit to hospital for X-rays. An ambulance was called and arrived promptly. On arrival at the hospital, Danny was in a great deal of pain, assumed to be from his ankle injury, and the nurses tried to make him comfortable while the doctor dealt with some other patients. After about 20 minutes the doctor arrived and sent Danny for an X-ray of his ankle. While in the X-ray department, Danny became unresponsive and died within half an hour. Danny's post-mortem report showed massive abdominal bleeding from a ruptured spleen. He also had a fracture to his ankle.

There are important messages to learn from Danny's story.

- All injuries have the potential to be life- or limb-threatening.
- It is essential that problems are anticipated, rather than reacted to once they develop.

Activity 10.1   *Critical thinking*

- What assessment should have been carried out in Danny's case?
- What are you looking for in such an assessment, and why?

There is an outline answer to this activity at the end of the chapter.

The primary survey

The objective of this phase is to identify and correct any immediately life-threatening conditions, including the airway, breathing, circulation, disability and exposure (ABCDE). To do this, the activities in Table 10.1 need to be carried out. The survey follows a simple mnemonic of A, B, C, D, E. These should be worked through in sequence and any issues resolved before proceeding to the next stage of the survey.

On admission to the emergency department the ATLS assessment will primarily be the physician's responsibility. However, all members of the team should be able to contribute to patient safety by having their own awareness of the framework in use. When the primary survey has been completed it should be repeated before proceeding to the secondary survey in order to ensure that new problems have not arisen and that nothing important has been missed.

The secondary survey

Once life-threatening conditions have been treated, or excluded, then you can carry out the secondary survey. This is a comprehensive head-to-toe examination of the patient, which provides the basis of the admission documentation. You need to pay close attention to the history

Airway and control of cervical spine	Must be considered in conjunction with each other as interventions performed on the airway will impact on the c-spine and vice versa. E.g. if you need to perform an emergency intubation for the patient and utilise the usual head-tilt, then you may lose control of the c-spine with catastrophic results. (Jaw thrust should be used until c-spine is cleared.) Similarly, intubating the already triply immobilised patient presents its own challenges for the anaesthetist and assisting staff. Intubation would be indicated where respiration is absent, where GCS <8 or electively where smoke inhalation, oral burns or facial trauma present risks to the airway from gross oedema that may narrow and distort the airway.
Breathing	Normal oxygenation and respiration is the aim. Note rate, depth of respirations and listen for normal breath sounds. How is the gas exchange? You may be able to make a quick assumption of this initially from signs of cyanosed skin or laboured breathing although urgent arterial blood gas confirmation will be required. Remember, carbon monoxide poisoning may give the patient a cherry red complexion, and saturations may appear normal as carbon monoxide binds to haemoglobin. Full-thickness circumferential burns to the chest may cause restriction of breathing mechanically.
Circulation	Establishing reliable venous access is a priority at this point in order to carry out any subsequent treatment as you continue with your primary survey. Delays in gaining venous access may make obtaining access more problematic as the patient progresses into shock. Diagnostic blood tests should be taken for full blood count, coagulation, cross match, electrolytes. Arterial blood gas analysis and, where appropriate, carboxyhaemoglobin levels would provide interim information until formal blood results are available. Haemorrhage control should be established and treatment for shock initiated with fluid resuscitation. Examination of chest, abdomen and pelvis should be carried out at this stage.
Disability	Patient responsiveness should be assessed using the GCS and examination of pupil reaction. Blood sugar measurements should be taken at this time.
Exposure	The patient should be undressed for a full body examination, but hypothermia must also be prevented. If possible, thoracic and lumbar spine should be cleared at this stage. Any wounds should be assessed for further management.

Table 10.1: The primary survey

of this accident and of previous medical history so that important details that may suggest other injuries or complicating factors are not overlooked. You will take a detailed history of the accident from the patient, witnesses, relatives, GP or medical alert jewellery, if worn. If attending paramedics are present, it is essential to gain information from them before they leave (Cole, 2009).

The mnemonic AMPLE helps you to remember what information you need to obtain during the assessment.

- **A**llergies.
- **M**edication.
- **P**ast medical history.
- **L**ast meal/fluid.
- **E**vents relevant to injury.

The secondary survey should revisit all elements of the primary survey in ABCDE priority order, and you should pay attention to important information that may have had to be deferred while the primary survey was establishing the basis of patient survival.

The secondary survey is one of time and detail as an in-depth assessment of each body region is warranted. You must monitor vital signs, and examine your patient's head/skull for irregularity or scalp wound, check the ears for blood or CSF leaks, and check eyes for pupil size and reaction (PEARL – Pupils Equal and Reactive to Light). Observe the thorax for bruising and possible fracture. All four limbs need to be checked for irregularity, deformity and fractures; compare limbs with each other and look for shortening and rotation. Finally, the patient's back needs to be checked for fracture and any spinal irregularities. Logrolling should be adopted until the c-spine is cleared by the physicians and documented in the medical notes. Once the primary and secondary surveys have been completed by the medical team, unconscious or confused patients in particular are generally reliant on the nurse to anticipate and identify any deterioration in their condition. Thus the principles of the primary survey ABCDE can be utilised in everyday practice to provide structure to your own assessment of the patient.

Activity 10.2   *Reflection*

Think back to your experiences in the clinical setting and identify examples of situations of when you had to complete a primary survey and a secondary survey.

- In the primary survey, what were the main priorities for the patient and why?
- In the secondary survey, what clinical signs and features were present and did this affect your prioritisation of care?

Hint: These reflective questions will help you to practise linking the importance of treating problems as they are found. The ABCDE order of treatment reflects the importance of treatment priority.

There is no outline answer at the end of the chapter as this activity is based on your own reflections.

Before moving on to each section of the secondary survey, remember to go back and keep checking the patient's ABCs. Avoid the common error of being distracted before the whole body has been inspected, as potentially serious injuries can be missed, especially in the unconscious patient. For example, the clinical staff may have noted that the patient was wearing rings that were compromising the circulation to the digits during the primary survey, but this would be of little consequence if the patient was not breathing at that time.

In the next section we will consider the clinical features of the metabolic response to trauma and we will explore how you can assess and manage the patient in order to provide clinically effective care.

Metabolic response to trauma

When the body sustains a traumatic injury, an inflammatory response starts from the site of tissue damage as chemical mediators are released. (Mediators are signalling chemical molecules involved in transmitting information between cells.)

The **inflammatory mediators** involved are:

* **histamine**;
* **kinins** (polypeptides);
* **prostaglandins** (fatty acids);
* **leukotrienes**.

All of these mediators in turn cause vasodilation and subsequently increased blood flow, which brings phagocytes and leukocytes to the original injury to deal with infections or foreign agents and to begin repairing the injury. **Vascular permeability** is enhanced by the mediators, which in turn permit clotting proteins such as fibrin, the enzymatic serum protein complement, kinins and white blood cells to reach the tissue.

Once the clotting proteins have moved from the blood into the tissues, an osmotic change occurs and oedema forms in the tissue at the site of injury. The clotting proteins then isolate any abnormal agents such as particles or bacteria at the source of the injury by forming an encasing clot to isolate it from the surrounding normal tissue.

Now let us consider some minor trauma, which will make it easier for you to understand how the body responds to major trauma.

Case study

*Lily, a hardworking student nurse, has decided to attend a ward night out. She has been saving for some lovely shoes, which don't really fit properly but look fantastic. As the evening progresses, the shoes start to rub her heels and they begin to look red. Lily realises that the trauma she is experiencing is **abrasive trauma**.*

Lily is not in a position to change her shoes so they continue to rub until a blister starts to form as fluid leaks into the tissues from the vasodilation that the inflammatory mediators cause as they rush to the injured area. The pain she experiences is caused by localised swelling from the inflammatory response and by mechanical means as the shoes continue to rub. Eventually, the blister breaks, leaving an open wound and a portal for bacterial entry. Nerve endings are now exposed as the top of the blister bursts, causing further pain.

Monitoring the critically ill patient

The critical care setting can be a daunting environment to those unfamiliar with caring for such sick patients. Many pieces of previously unseen equipment are in use for monitoring and treating the patient: for example, blood pressure may be recorded continuously on-screen via an arterial line, giving a blood pressure that varies from beat to beat rather than via a cuff measurement that gives a random, one-off blood pressure reading. Many patients will be assisted with bodily functions that are normally autonomic such as breathing or renal filtration by machinery. Multiple intravenous infusions may be in progress at the same time.

However, as with the patient's initial assessment after injury, the primary survey can be adapted and should be continuously revisited by the nurse caring for the patient in order to ensure the safety of the patient. Once the primary and secondary survey has been completed by the medical team, unconscious or confused patients in particular are generally reliant on the nurse to anticipate and identify any deterioration in their condition.

Activity 10.3   *Reflection*

Think back to your experiences in a critical care clinical setting.

- How did you deal with major trauma in a critical care setting and what were your nursing priorities with regard to care delivery and best practice?

These reflective questions will help you prioritise your patient care through examining the means of clinically monitoring and continuously assessing the major trauma patient.

There is no outline answer at the end of the chapter as this activity is based on your own reflections.

Case study

Mrs Sharon Bowen, aged 25, sustained a 60% flame burn to her upper body from a witnessed suicide attempt in her parked car after suffering from post-natal depression. She was intubated by the paramedics, and 100% oxygen was administered prior to arrival at A&E as smoke contains dangerous gases such as carbon monoxide that need to be addressed by administering high concentrations of oxygen even before confirmation from blood results (Herndon, 2007).

The c-spine had not been immobilised as Mrs Bowen's accident did not involve any impact and the witnesses to the accident were able to state the mechanism of the injury. Lily, the student, is on duty when Mrs Bowen arrives. She observes the primary survey being undertaken by the medical and nursing staff.

Airway *is deemed to be patent following intubation.* Breathing *is occurring with assistance, but bagging the patient is difficult and the chest is not rising much with each breath delivered. Arterial blood gas analysis reveals significant respiratory and metabolic acidosis. Lily notes that Mrs Bowen's trunk is burned circumferentially, and the anaesthetist explains that this is why it is difficult to ventilate the patient. An emergency* **escharotomy** *is performed on the spot by the doctors to release the taut burned skin that is restricting chest movement. This involves making an incision with a sterile blade through the depth of the burned tissue and extending into unburned skin. This results in an immediate improvement in chest expansion as the patient is easier to bag, with better oxygenation and gas exchange evident on the next arterial blood gas. From this, Lily realises that a secured airway does not automatically mean that the patient will be able to breathe: steps need to be taken to ensure that breathing can take place, such as bagging to manually inflate the chest or addressing other complicating factors, in this case the deep burns to the chest, making bagging difficult and requiring emergency intervention. Escharotomies are performed under general anaesthetic except in an emergency situation such as this where time delays could mean that the patient will not survive.*

Mrs Bowen's arterial blood gases were as follows.

continued . . .

Prior to escharotomy	1 hour post escharotomy
pH 7.05 pCO_2 9.0kPa pO_2 10.5kPa	pH 7.30 pCO_2 7.0kPa pO_2 14kPa

Note the rapid improvement in Mrs Bowen's arterial blood gases following escharotomy once she is able to fully expand her chest and exhale carbon dioxide more efficiently. While the blood gases have not yet reached normality, you will recognise a significant improvement from the earlier blood gas analysis.

Blood gas analysis may be measured in millimetres of mercury or kilopascals depending on the blood gas analyser (see Table 10.2).

Kilopascal measurements	Millimetres of mercury measurement
pH 7.35–7.45 pO_2 11.5–13.5kPa pCO_2 4.5–6kPa HCO_3 25–30mmol/L Base excess −2 to +2	pH 7.35–7.45 pO_2 80–100mmHg pCO_2 35–45mmHg HCO_3 25–30mmol/L Base excess −2 to +2

Table 10.2: Normal values for arterial blood gases

Only once the airway, breathing and cervical spine elements of the primary survey have been addressed, should consideration be given to the other elements of the primary survey such as circulation, disability and exposure. Initially, the circulation component of the survey will be concerned with checking that the pulse is present and noting whether it is strong and bounding or weak and thread. Then capillary refill can be checked by applying pressure to an area of skin (unburned area in this patient). The skin should blanch and return to normal within two seconds. If it does not, then you may have a hypovolaemic patient.

However, other limbs should be tested in order to exclude a localised problem with the circulation. For example, if the limb has a circumferential burn, circulation may be sluggish locally but fine generally. Excluding the possibility of major haemorrhage is the immediate priority. Establishing venous access, while important, should not come before first aid for bleeding. Direct pressure should be applied where serious bleeding occurs. Commencing intravenous fluid resuscitation can be dealt with during the secondary survey, provided access has already been established. If access cannot be gained intravenously, then intraosseous access may have to be considered. When these have been addressed, other factors such as disability can be considered. As Mrs Bowen has already been intubated, this could prove to be difficult as the normal AVPU measures of Alertness, Vocal Stimulus, Response to Painful Stimuli and Unresponsiveness may be affected by sedatives. However, the aim is to exclude signs of head injury and maxillofacial trauma, and in this situation pupil reaction to light would need to be assessed before proceeding to complete exposure of the patient in order to ensure that no other life-threatening injuries have been missed. Care must be taken to keep the patient warm during this part of the assessment. If a warm environment cannot be provided, then the patient may have to be exposed in stages to prevent hypothermia. Jewellery should be removed and kept safe at this stage.

With all forms of major trauma, regardless of cause, the risk of hypovolaemic shock is present, along with sepsis either from the original injury or the invasive devices used to monitor the patient's condition. These risk factors may perpetuate the inflammatory response in a negative way, so that it moves from being beneficial to becoming detrimental to the patient.

Activity 10.4   *Decision-making*

- In this situation what things can be overlooked?

There is an outline answer to this question at the end of the chapter

---

Case study

Mr David Jones is a 31-year-old man who sustained a crush injury to his abdomen from heavy machinery at work. Primary and secondary surveys are conducted in A&E and he is taken straight to theatre to explore an open abdominal wound. Lily, the student, is working under supervision with her mentor who is allocated as Mr Jones's nurse when he arrives from theatre. He has multiple injuries including pelvic fractures. The peritoneum has been found to be intact but a vacuum-assisted closure (VAC) drain is in situ due to a large surface of skin loss over the abdomen with a small but steady drainage of **haemoserous fluid**. *On arrival from theatre Mr Jones's vital signs are remarkably stable. He appears pale, but he is prescribed a further two units of red blood cells post-operatively that were not completed in theatre, and these are in the process of being ordered. He has intravenous fluid running and a patient-controlled analgesia (PCA) pump for analgesia but is not dependent on inotropic support. Mr Jones's family have been spoken to by the surgeon as Mr Jones remains on a ventilator in ITU. Her mentor starts the admission paperwork after setting up the first unit of blood. As Lily begins to document the patient's observations, the VAC begins to alarm.*

Lily checks the cause of the alarm and notices that the 1 litre VAC chamber has completely filled with frank blood. Mr Jones remains pale but otherwise does not appear to have deteriorated drastically. His heart rate has increased a little and he is now mildly tachycardic. Blood pressure is not yet affected. Lily draws the mentor's attention to the situation. Another nurse is asked to contact the medical staff as Lily and her mentor reassess the patient.

Using the primary survey as a framework, Lily realises that airway *and* breathing *are secure and stable as Mr Jones remains on the ventilator but is able to initiate his own breaths. There is a slight rise in respiratory rate from 16 previously to 24 breaths per minute.* Circulation *has become a concern due to the blood loss into the VAC, and closer inspection of the patient reveals a significant amount of blood into the bed underneath the patient, although the abdominal dressing does not appear unduly saturated with blood as the fluid has leaked downwards under the dressing as the patient has been lying in a semi-recumbent position. Lily realises the importance of* exposure *of the patient as one of the components of the primary survey as some issues may not be obvious initially. As the medical staff arrive, Mr Jones becomes hypotensive with a blood pressure of 83/50. After checking an arterial blood gas measurement, which reveals a haemoglobin level of 6.8 and slight metabolic acidosis, the medical staff request that the unit of blood in progress is given at a faster rate and the*

continued . . .

next unit is ordered immediately. Arrangements are made for Mr Jones to return to theatre for exploration of the source of the bleeding. Mr Jones returns from theatre before the end of the shift. The second surgery identifies that a small artery in the existing abdominal wound was bleeding. This was repaired and Mr Jones made good progress, culminating in his discharge from the critical care unit several days later.

Activity 10.5   *Critical thinking*

- With reference to the case study, what clinical signs would indicate that Mr Jones's condition was getting worse?
- What could be the possible causes for his metabolic acidosis?

There is an outline answer to this activity at the end of the chapter

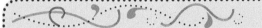

Chapter summary

The aim of this chapter was to help you to assess, recognise and respond to patients who sustain physiological trauma. In this chapter we have focused on the assessment and management of primary and secondary surveys and the metabolic response to trauma. In all of the clinical examples illustrated the key responsibilities of the nurse are the same.

- The ABCDE order of treatment reflects the differing things that can go wrong for trauma patients.
- Problems are treated as they are found – if a problem is found and treated and the patient deteriorates, you start again and work through ABCDE.
- Knowledge about a pattern of injury is helpful as a discovery of one injury should prompt you to search for a related injury.

Activities: brief outline answers

Activity 10.1: Critical thinking (page 186)

Missed intra-abdominal injuries and concealed haemorrhage are frequent causes of increased morbidity and mortality, especially in patients who survive the initial phase after an injury. Danny's abdomen should have been exposed and examined during the primary/secondary survey, which was not completed as Danny did not appear to have life-threatening injuries. Inspection of the abdomen would have revealed distension associated with bleeding and may have saved his life.

Activity 10.4: Decision-making (page 192)

Things that can be overlooked in this situation are airway burns, major trauma and inhalation exposure to carbon dioxide. Mrs Bowen's scenario represents a textbook situation in which the principles of the ATLS have been utilised to their full potential. Mrs Bowen will remain very ill for many more weeks, but giving the patient the best possible start on their road to recovery begins at the scene of the accident and continues through the emergency unit and onto specialist services such as the burns centre.

Activity 10.5: Critical thinking (page 193)

Mr Jones would have an increased respiratory rate, increased heart rate and decreasing blood pressure as the body attempts to compensate for the sudden blood loss.

The main cause of his metabolic acidosis would be hypovolaemia due to the excessive hydrogen ions produced in shock.

Mr Jones's story demonstrated to Lily the importance of checking a patient thoroughly (exposure), and she also learned how quickly a seemingly stable patient can deteriorate after major trauma and major surgery. It is essential to keep utilising the principles of the primary and secondary surveys even when a patient may seem to be on the road to recovery.

Further reading

Bosworth, C (2003) *Burns trauma: management and nursing care*, 2nd edition. London: Bailliere Tindall.

This book considers the treatment needs of patients of all ages with different types of burn injury, in a variety of clinical environments, and it is a valuable resource for all grades of staff within the multi-disciplinary team caring for patients with burn injuries.

Edwards, M and Griffiths, P (2011) *Emergency nursing made incredibly easy*. Philadelphia PA: Lippincott, Williams and Wilkins.

This book covers emergency care basics including patient assessment and triage, trauma, disease crises, and patient and family communication, as well as legal issues such as handling evidence and documentation and holistic issues such as pain and end-of-life care. It offers essential information on emergency, trauma and critical care in an easy-to-follow format.

Mackway-Jones, K, Marsden, J and Windle J (2006*) Manchester triage group. Emergency triage*, 2nd edition. Oxford: Blackwell Publishing.

This practical handbook will be an essential purchase for all health service staff who deal with emergencies. It guides the user through the basic methodology of triage, and then demonstrates how to apply the principles of all the major emergency presentation using easy-to-follow flow charts.

Useful websites

www.nice.org.uk/

This website allows you to access a series of national clinical guidelines to secure consistent, high-quality, evidence-based care for patients using the National Health Service.

www.who.int/publications/en

This is an easy, user-friendly website that provides summaries of the best available evidence relating to best practice and supporting policy.

Chapter 11
Patients and relatives with psychological trauma

Desiree Tait with Bethan James

continued . . .

By entry to the register:

xii. Acts with dignity and respect to ensure that people who are unable to meet their activities of living have choices about how these are met and feel empowered to do as much as possible for themselves.

xiii. Works autonomously, confidently and in partnership with people, their families and carers to ensure that needs are met through care planning and delivery, including strategies for self-care and peer support.

Chapter aims

By the end of this chapter, you should be able to:

- identify factors that positively and negatively affect patients and their relatives during a period of critical illness;
- demonstrate an awareness of how the impact of critical illness can be felt by patients and relatives following their discharge from intensive care;
- describe how the psychological needs of patients and relatives may be met by the nurse and health care team;
- demonstrate an awareness of the psychological and emotional work involved in caring for critically ill patients and their families.

Introduction: the psychological impact of being a patient in intensive care

When patients become critically ill and they, with their family, enter the intensive care unit (ICU), the physiological and psychological impact can be far-reaching, regardless of the patients' outcomes, and can still affect the well-being of the patients and/or their families for years after the event. In the story below, Sally is invited to reflect on her experience as a patient in critical care.

Case study: Sally's story

When I was 19 years old I had meningitis and septicaemia. It happened during my first term at university and they said that if it hadn't been for the swift action of my flatmates, I would have died. I was very drowsy and can only remember lying on my bed in the residences, so my parents explained some of what happened later but, to be honest, I didn't want to know. According to Mum, I stayed in the ICU for five days and was eventually well enough to go home after another week in hospital.

One year on, apart from my nightmares that involve me falling into a noisy waterfall and choking, I thought I was over it completely. That was until I was contacted by a nurse researcher who asked if she could interview

continued . . .

me about my illness. I said that I couldn't remember being in ICU but agreed to be interviewed as long as I didn't have to go to the hospital. Visits to the hospital would always seem to trigger headaches that would last for days so I tended to avoid hospitals if I could.

During the interview I began to recount my experience, and suddenly it was as if I was transported back to that time and place. I was naked and vulnerable, terrified and abused. I was choking in a waterfall. I wanted to shout 'stop' but no sound came out. I tried to get out and run away, but I was tied down and my arms and legs felt so heavy. Then I saw Mum's face and she held me. I could remember Mum and Dad holding my hand and the nurse always being there – I didn't have to call her.

I hadn't realised until that interview how traumatised I had felt and how I had unwittingly pushed the memories to the back of my mind, too painful to recall. In a way the interview helped, and now I am learning to understand and cope with the bad and good memories of intensive care. I have asked for more details of the time, and now I know that the waterfall was the noise of the suction when they cleared secretions from my throat. I thought they were trying to kill me!

What Sally's story tells us is that being a patient in ICU can be frightening, especially when you have no idea of how and why you are there. In this chapter we will explore the psychological impact of critical illness on the patient from its onset through to the rehabilitation and/or discharge. A critically ill patient experiences not only physiological trauma, but also a range of emotions and memories that can trigger long-term psychological trauma for both the patient and family, regardless of the patient's outcome (Pattison, 2005; Kiekkas et al., 2010; Samuelson, 2011).

In the first section we will examine Sally's story in more detail and explore some of the factors that influenced her experience of being in ICU.

Why did Sally have such a sudden reaction to being asked to tell her story?

The reaction Sally had when asked to recall her experiences is a manifestation of the psychological trauma she experienced during her critical illness and stay in ICU. There are four main factors that influenced the development of her psychological distress.

- *The suddenness and acuteness of her illness*: Sally described being away at university where the stress and exposure of a new environment would have made her susceptible to infection. She was immunised against *Haemophilus influenzae* type b (Hib) bacterial meningitis, but this still left her exposed to other strains of the disease (Kennedy, 2009). The onset of the infection was rapid: over the course of an evening she went from feeling as though she had a cold to being semiconscious. She was unconscious when she arrived in ICU and only began to wake up 48 hours later. As she regained consciousness she found herself in an alien environment with unfamiliar sounds, lighting and people, and she was terrified.
- *The medication she required*: Sally was prescribed intravenous antibiotics, pain relief in the form of an opioid and sedation to treat the infection and support effective mechanical ventilation and cerebral perfusion. All these drugs are known to trigger delirium in the critically ill patient

(see Table 8.2 on pages 154–5). Sally was prescribed **midazolam**, a short-acting sedative of the group **benzodiazepine**, and this would have affected her ability to rationalise and remember information. As a consequence, Sally would have felt as though she was in a dream world, unable to focus on what was happening and why, or to remember it.

- *Neurological, cardiovascular and circulatory instability related to bacterial meningitis and sepsis*: The physiological impact of Sally's illness led to a state of altered consciousness, fever, hypoxia, fluctuations in blood pressure and fluid, and electrolyte imbalance. These physiological factors are all known to trigger the onset of confusion, anxiety and delirium (Arend and Christensen, 2009).
- *Loss of control of verbal communication and independent mobility due to the presence of invasive monitoring and therapy*: In ICU Sally was intubated with an oral endotracheal tube (ETT) tied around her face and neck and attached to ventilator tubing. The ETT passes via the vocal cords into the trachea, meaning that Sally was unable to communicate verbally. Other invasive equipment would have included an arterial line, central venous line, naso-gastric tube and urinary catheter. Less invasive monitoring equipment attached to Sally included technology to measure oxygen saturation and cardiac monitoring. Sally would have felt weighed down by the equipment and frightened by the strange noises and environment. She would be weak from her illness and unable to call for help. Her experience is illustrated in Figure 11.1.

When Sally tried to recall her illness it triggered memories of frightening events, anxiety and distress that she had managed to suppress from her waking hours until she experienced a flashback to an event during the interview. In her story Sally describes trying to shout for help and run away. She described feeling naked and vulnerable, and feeling as though she was choking. When Sally reflected back on the experience with her parents, this feeling of terror related to when the nurse aspirated secretions from her endotracheal tube. Sally felt naked because she was naked, apart from a small sheet covering her modesty, as the nurses tried to reduce her fever. Sally's description is consistent with a response to extreme fear and relates to the responses of freeze (hyper-vigilance), flight, fight and fright (tonic immobility) described by Gray (1987). Sally

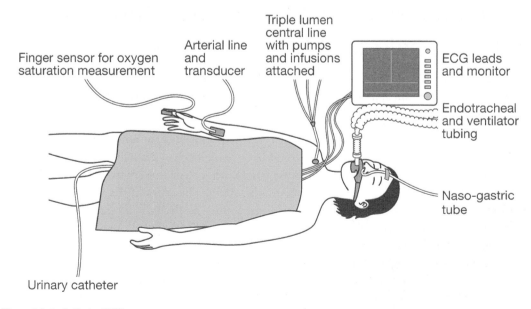

Figure 11.1: Sally in ICU

– hyper-vigilant and responsive to the danger even in her sedated state – tried to run away but found herself trapped by her own physical weakness and the monitoring equipment.

The symptoms and feelings Sally experienced can be described as post-traumatic stress disorder (PTSD) associated with her experience of being critically ill in ICU. The symptoms of PTSD are either specific to the trauma and involve flash-backs and avoidance of triggers, or are manifested as hyper-arousal and anxiety. Three symptom groups associated with PTSD are set out in Table 11.1 and relate to Sally's story (American Psychiatric Association, 2004; Smith and Segal, 2011).

Sally's story illustrates that the trauma and anxiety related to critical illness can affect a patient's recovery and rehabilitation. Research into the psychological implications of critical illness has demonstrated consistently that patients in ICU and their families experience anxiety both during and following discharge, as well as acute stress disorder (PTSD), depression and lethargy (Pattison, 2005; Kiekkas et al., 2010). According to Samuelson (2011), these negative feelings can be counterbalanced with memories that reinforce safety, trust and having a sense of control. Often when patients are discharged from ICU their anxieties and distress continue. One manifestation of this is transfer anxiety or relocation stress, and has been shown to affect both patients and their families. The story below illustrates an example of a patient and his family's experience of relocation anxiety.

Symptom group	Common symptoms	Sally's symptoms
Re-experiencing the trauma event	• Intrusive and upsetting memories of the event. • Flashbacks (feeling like the event is repeating). • Nightmares. • Feelings of intense distress when reminded of the traumatic event. • Physiological stress response when reminded of the event.	• Flashbacks: Suddenly it was as if I was transported back to that time and place. I was naked and vulnerable, terrified and abused. • I was choking in a waterfall, I wanted to shout stop but no sound came out. • My arms and legs felt too heavy and I couldn't run away. • Nightmares: I had a recurring nightmare that involved me falling into a noisy waterfall and choking. • Headaches when visiting the hospital. • I thought they were trying to kill me.
Avoidance and numbing	• Avoiding anything that reminds you of the trauma. • Unable to remember significant aspects of the event. • Loss of interest in life, general lethargy. • Feeling detached and emotionally numb. • Sense of having a limited future; awareness of your own limited mortality.	• It happened during my first term at university; my parents explained some of what happened later but to be honest I didn't want to know. • Subsequent visits to the hospital always seem to trigger headaches that would last for days so I tended to avoid hospitals if I could. • I haven't gone back to university yet, perhaps next year if I'm still alive.

Table 11.1: Symptoms of PTSD related to Sally's story

Continued

Symptom group	Common symptoms	Sally's symptoms
Increased anxiety and emotional arousal	• Difficulty with sleeping, not being able to fall asleep or waking early. • Difficulty with concentration. • Outbursts of anger, irritability. • Being hyper-vigilant. • Feeling jumpy and easily startled.	• Woken by the nightmares. • I don't like going too far from home.

Table 11.1: Continued

Case study: Brian Smith

Brian is a 58-year-old executive who, prior to hospitalisation, smoked three cigars a day. Three weeks ago Brian collapsed at work with severe back pain; he required emergency surgery for a leaking abdominal aortic aneurism. Brian required invasive ventilation for eight days after surgery, for treatment of pneumonia and severe sepsis, and a further six days of close monitoring as he was weaned from respiratory and haemodynamic support. When, on Friday afternoon, Brian and his wife Helen were told he was ready for discharge to the ward they felt elated as this meant he was a step closer to recovery. Brian was subsequently transferred within an hour of being given the information, as there was an emergency and they needed the bed.

Within an hour of Brian's transfer Helen began to get upset because Brian was in a cubicle away from the other patients; he was not on a monitor and there were only two registered nurses to cover the whole ward. She was frightened that no one was looking after him. The ward had restricted visiting, and Helen was only able to visit for short periods twice a day. After a few hours on the ward Brian also became anxious and frightened because he couldn't see any nurses. He started to press the call button every 30 minutes so that he could see and talk to someone and feel reassured. The nurses and health care support workers did not, however, offer much reassurance and rarely stayed for more than a minute. Brian began to lose his trust in them and refused his food and medication, frightened that they were trying to poison him. He became very agitated and tried to run away from the ward. The following day his condition had deteriorated further and he was readmitted to ICU. Helen said, 'I knew this would happen.'

Why did Brian develop transfer anxiety and how did this impact on his rehabilitation?

Carpenito (2000, p715) defines relocation stress as: 'a state in which an individual experiences physiologic and/or psychological disturbances as a result of transfer from one environment to another'. This condition has been highlighted by Chaboyer et al. (2005) as a common occurrence when patients are transferred from a one-to-one nursing environment to a ward where they are expected to take on a more independent role in their recovery and rehabilitation.

When Brian's care was reviewed, there appeared to be three main factors that led to him experiencing relocation stress, which delayed his rehabilitation and led to a second admission to ICU. These were as follows.

- *Length of stay in ICU*: Brian was a patient in ICU for 14 days, the first eight of which he was intubated and ventilated. He was then gradually weaned from respiratory support, and by the time he was transferred to the ward he was breathing unaided with the support of 28% oxygen. The longer the length of time a patient remains critically ill, the greater the risk of them developing delirium and psychological problems such as anxiety, nightmares and problems with sleeping. It is important to assess the patient for any signs of psychological distress and to be aware of the risk factors associated with the onset of delirium (see Chapter 8).

- *Transfer from an environment where there was a patient-to-nurse ratio of 1:1 to an environment with a ratio of 12:1*: ICU patients such as Brian often feel abandoned, vulnerable and unimportant when they are transferred to a ward (Chaboyer et al., 2005). Brian was the centre of attention for 14 days with one-to-one nursing care; he felt safe and cared for. The sudden transition to being one of 12 patients being cared for by one nurse was a clear contrast and one that he felt unable to cope with. He had never met any of the ward staff and had an overwhelming sense of vulnerability and helplessness. The ward nurses were working to their maximum capabilities, but Brian began to feel an overwhelming sense of panic. When Brian's wife expressed her concern about the reduction in the level of care on the ward, this added to his anxieties, and both he and his wife became mistrusting of the ward staff.

- *No evidence of a structured discharge and rehabilitation plan*: Brian was transferred at short notice, and the ward staff were unprepared for his admission. ICU needed a bed for an emergency patient and Brian was assessed by the medical team as being well enough to be transferred. During his time in ICU, the staff had focused on the day-to-day management of Brian's care. When he was transferred the staff gave a comprehensive review of Brian's physiological care provision but had not included an assessment of his psychological state. Part of the handover had included a summary of information given to the family about Brian's prognosis, but no goals or targets had been set for his rehabilitation. In situations where a patient transfer has been hurried, both ward staff and patients can be apprehensive about the process. This process is often complicated by the large amount of documentation and information that comes with the patient and a lack of understanding by the ward staff about what the patient has experienced. Conversely, the high expectations of the patient with regard to the level of care they will receive add stress and strain to the nurse–patient relationship even before the nurse has a chance to get to know the patient (Beard, 2005).

Poor quality rehabilitation and follow-up after discharge from intensive care has been identified as a factor that can lead to increased patient morbidity. The response by the National Institute for Health and Clinical Excellence (NICE, 2009) was to publish a clinical guideline on rehabilitation after critical illness. The guideline proposes that patients should receive five phases of bio-psychosocial assessment and support. These should occur:

1. during the patient's time in ICU;
2. prior to discharge from ICU;
3. during ward-based care;
4. prior to discharge into the community;
5. two to three months following discharge from ICU.

They go on to suggest that there should be continuity of care during the rehabilitation programme so that recovery and rehabilitation is seen as the continuous and inevitable outcome of critical care rather than the exception. When Brian was transferred to the ward, it appeared that all links with the intensive care team were lost, and this added to his sense of abandonment. In 2003 the Department of Health with the NHS Modernisation Agency published guidance on the development of outreach services that would:

- support ward staff with the recognition and fast tracking of patients with clinical deterioration to effective clinical management;
- provide ongoing support and monitoring of patients recently discharged from ICU.

This and the NICE guidance (2009) suggest that a structured and collaborative approach to discharge together with continuity of patient care can facilitate a holistic and patient-centred rehabilitation with the potential for reduced morbidity following critical illness.

Brian's anxiety and his refusal to take diet, fluids and medication led to a deterioration in his medical condition. He became dehydrated, hypotensive and hypoxic. As a result, he was readmitted to ICU where he received respiratory, fluid and electrolyte resuscitation. Brian was eventually discharged from ICU to the ward 48 hours later. He was visited by staff from the unit every day until he felt reassured that he was safe once more and his condition continued to improve. A week later he was discharged home with the support of the community team with an appointment to see the critical care liaison nurse four weeks from hospital discharge.

Activity 11.1   *Reflection*

The purpose of this reflection is not to find a right or wrong answer but to help you to develop your self-awareness of the factors that may influence how you now assess and manage bio-psychosocial aspects of care, and how that may change in the future.

Think back to your experiences in the clinical setting and patients you have nursed. Can you remember caring for patients who you would describe as difficult or challenging in their behaviour towards you or the staff on the ward? If so, write a description of the events and reflect on the following.

- Was the patient admitted as an emergency?
- Was the patient transferred from a critical care area?
- What type of challenging behaviour did the patient or family display?
- Now try to think of physical, psychological or socio-cultural factors that may have influenced their behaviour.
- How was their care managed and was it successful?
- Were their other strategies to manage their care that could have been used?

As this activity is for your own reflection, there is no answer at the end of the chapter.

What are the needs of the families of critically ill patients?

In Brian's story, his wife Helen had experienced a chaos of emotions since she was informed of his collapse by the personnel department where Brian worked. She had gone from feeling safe and reassured by her daily routine to feeling threatened and traumatised because of her husband's collapse. Helen entered a period of confusion and high anxiety, waiting anxiously for the outcome of the surgery and Brian's stay in ICU. Hopkins (1994) describes patients and their families experiencing a pattern of feelings and emotions akin to grief and loss, with families going through stages of adjustment until they are able to come to terms with the situation. This is illustrated in Figure 11.2 with Helen's experiences described in the boxes.

The psychological needs of families during critical illness have been a subject of intensive research that began with Molter's (1979) validation of the Critical Care Family Needs Inventory (CCFNI). During the last 20 years the CCFNI has been tested for validity and reliability and updated to reflect an increased emphasis on developing family-centred care (Kinrade et al., 2009). The needs of families have been shown to focus on five core categories and include the provision of:

- information;
- the ability to be near the patient;
- reassurance;
- support;
- comfort.

According to Kinrade et al. (2009) the five most important itemised needs of families in these categories are:

1. to have questions answered honestly;
2. to be able to visit any time;
3. to feel that the hospital personnel care about the patient;

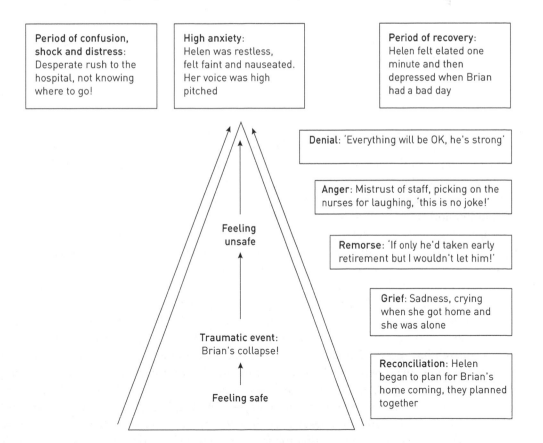

Figure 11.2: Phases of psychological crisis for Helen and its manifestations

203

4. to know specific facts concerning the patient's progress;
5. to know the expected outcome.

In Brian and Helen's story these needs were sensitively met until the urgent requirement to transfer Brian meant that they did not received all the support and information necessary for Brian's transfer (Mitchell et al., 2003). As a consequence they were unprepared for the step down in the level of care received and the rules imposed with regard to restricted visiting. The sense of trust and safety they had felt in ICU had to be rebuilt with different nurses and different rules.

What can we do as nurses to reduce the risks associated with psychological trauma in critically ill patients and their families?

Nursing in the twenty-first century takes place in an environment where patient care relies on complex biomedical technology and therapy to support appropriate patient outcomes. Such technology and care can be delivered in patients' homes and in the hospital environment. The core element of nursing, however, remains unchanged, that is, to provide nursing care. Caring in the UK is core to the values of the code of practice that underpins nursing and is referred to 31 times in the *Code of conduct*, while the word 'professional ' is referred to only 14 times (NMC, 2008). Caring can be described as 'the human mode of being' (Roach, 1984, p2). Every human has the capacity to care; it is not exclusive to nursing but is essential to nursing (Boykin and Schoenhofer, 1993; Roach, 2002; Schoenhofer, 2001).

The challenge that we face as nurses is to recognise and demonstrate how caring can be seen and measured in nursing. In Figure 11.3, six key words from Roach's theory of nursing as caring – 'the six Cs' – show how in principle the elements of compassion, competence, confidence, conscience, commitment and comportment can be applied to patient and family needs and motivators, so that the negative feelings and behaviours of patients and families experiencing critical illness can be balanced with positive feelings and behaviours through the knowledge and skills of the nurse and health care team.

It is only by knowing and understanding the patient and family experience that we can begin to understand and support the patient and family towards an appropriate outcome. According to findings by Finfgeld-Connet (2007), caring is characterised by expert nursing practice, interpersonal sensitivity and intimate relationships. The quality of caring is determined by the patient's need for caring, and the nurse's professional maturity and ability to provide that care. In Table 11.2 the six Cs of caring have been applied in more detail to Brian and Helen's story in order to see how their psychological needs could have been met.

For you as a student, the knowledge and skills required to care for patients is developmental and will involve you developing expertise in the physical, psychological and socio-cultural aspects of care. Research has shown that students and qualified nurses often prioritise aspects of care differently. For some, the psychosocial aspects of care are the most important, such as touching the patient, listening and talking to them (Greenhalgh et al., 1998). For others it is the physical and safety aspects of care that are the most important (Kapborg, 2000; Khademian and Vizeshfar, 2007). Some research findings suggest that student nurses change their view of caring as they progress through the course, losing the idealised view of holistic caring and replacing it with professional and technical aspects of care (Mackintosh, 2006).

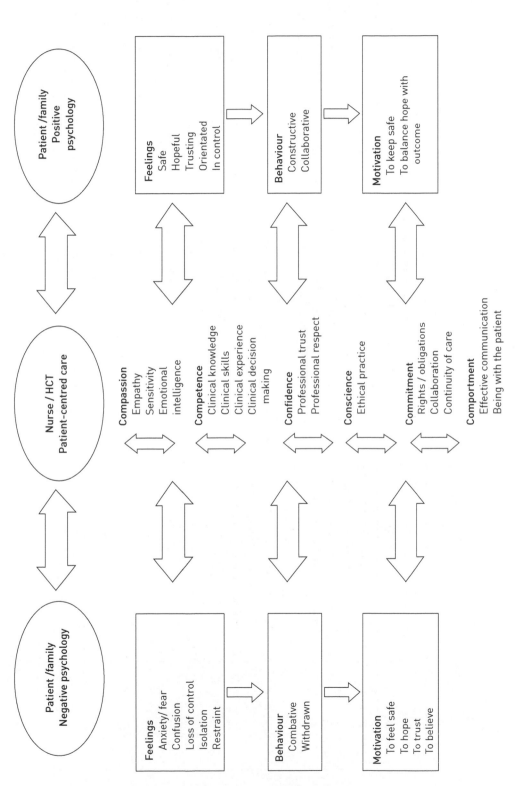

Figure 11.3: The role of the nurse and health care team (HCT) in facilitating positive patient and family psychology through patient-centred care

Caring theme	Objectives	Interventions to promote patient-centred care for Brian and Helen
Compassion	• To promote empathy and sensitivity to the patient and family's situation. • To respect the patient as an individual and their family as a social unit.	• Provide patient-centred care recognising Brian as an individual. • Utilise team nursing and a named nurse to manage continuity of care. • Keep a patient diary with the help of the family so that the patient can make sense of their time in ICU when they are able. • Provide support for Helen in the form of up-to-date information, booklets and updates on the patient's care.
Competence	• To demonstrate competence in the following clinical elements: knowledge; skills; experience; decision making.	• Provide a safe and holistic approach to care • Assess Brian and Helen for evidence of physical and psychological deterioration on each shift and communicate your findings. • Assess Brian for risk factors and signs of delirium on each shift and communicate your findings. • Promote and evaluate sleep and rest periods for Brian. • Plan for Brian's discharge and rehabilitation from the date of his admission. • Ensure that information given to Helen is up to date and documented in the patient's notes. • Provide a staged reduction in the continuous assessment and monitoring of Brian prior to discharge. • Provide an informed and comprehensive handover prior to and during Brian's discharge. • Negotiate plans for outreach and follow-up care.

Confidence	• To demonstrate trust and respect through confident and efficient practice.
Conscience	• To demonstrate ethical practice.
Commitment	• To demonstrate commitment by balancing the patient/family and nursing rights and obligations.
Comportment	• Demonstrate effective communication and being with the patient.

Confidence	• Demonstrate competence and confidence in the bio-psychosocial aspects of care. • Work in a collaborative manner with Brian, Helen and the health care team.
Conscience	• Be open and honest in all aspects of care. • Always act in Brian's best interest. • Encourage Brian and his family, if he agrees, to be involved in making ethical decisions.
Commitment	• Provide continuity of care. • Communicate the strengths and limitations of care with open honesty and develop realistic goals. • Work collaboratively with Brian and Helen to help them recognise their rights and obligations for progressing towards recovery.
Comportment	• Use verbal and non-verbal skills to ensure effective professional communication. • Give attention to Brian and Helen, demonstrate self-awareness and an authentic desire to care.

Table 11.2: Promoting patient-centred care for families and patients experiencing critical illness: Brian and Helen's story

Activity 11.2   *Reflection*

Again, the purpose of this reflection is not to find a right or wrong answer but to help you to develop your self-awareness of the factors that may influence how you prioritise bio-psychosocial aspects of care now, and how that may change in the future.

Think back to your experiences in the clinical setting and patients you have nursed.

- Was your priority for those patients physical, psychological or socio-cultural?
- Was it always the same order of priority, or different, depending on the patients' situations?
- Which of the factors below influenced your choice of prioritising the patients' caring needs?
  - Patient safety.
  - Patient behaviour (being noisy, aggressive, requesting help, being quiet, withdrawn).
  - Advice from other staff/mentor/educator.
  - Your feelings and emotions.
  - Your knowledge and understanding of the patient's situation.
  - Pressure from colleagues/senior staff.

As this activity is for your own reflection, there is no answer at the end of the chapter.

The emotional work of nursing and caring

Finally, we will consider some issues related to the emotional work involved in developing close professional relationships with patients and their families. The provision of a patient-centred and holistic approach to care requires that nurses give of themselves emotionally in the dynamic of the nurse/patient/family relationship (Henderson, 2002; Stayt, 2009). This type of work is described as emotional labour and is described in the concept summary.

Concept summary: Emotional labour

Emotional labour was described by Hochschild (1983, p246), 'as the induction or suppression of feeling to sustain an outward appearance that produces in others a sense of being cared for in a convivial safe place'. It is arguably the work involved in using and regulating expressions of emotions in nursing practice. In nursing this involves the initiation and establishment of the nurse/patient/family relationship. It involves the development of friendship, intimacy and trust within the boundaries of professional practice. In nursing this comes at an emotional cost, and studies have shown that nurses have developed distancing strategies to keep them emotionally safe. These include: focusing on physical tasks rather than facing the emotional task before them; using closed questioning techniques in order to bring the interaction to an end quickly; changing the subject or identifying another task that needs to be completed (Stayt, 2009). A more constructive approach involves the use of problem-based coping strategies that help nurses to interpret, understand and manage emotions in a clinically effective way.

How can we as nurses manage emotional labour?

In nursing the role emotions play in helping professionals think, make clinical decisions, find solutions and develop leadership potential has been recognised and valued (Beauvais et al., 2011; Smith, 2005). The skills required to manage this emotional work can be described as 'emotional intelligence'. Emotional intelligence requires of the nurse the ability to describe, examine and reason about emotions. According to Mayer et al. (1999) it is the ability to:

- perceive emotions;
- use emotions;
- understand emotions;
- manage emotions.

As a student you can begin to develop your own emotional intelligence through self-inquiry and reflection. The reflective activities in this chapter will help to trigger your thoughts about how you manage your emotions. You can think about your strengths and limitations, and begin to recognise your emotions and their impact on others. Think about your rights and obligations, your commitment to nursing and your motivation to practise as a nurse. Use them to reflect on your understanding of others and the interpersonal skills required to work collaboratively with patients, families and colleagues (Goleman, 1998).

Chapter summary

Within this chapter we have explored the psychological needs of patients and their families and explored ways in which we as nurses can help them to come to terms with the impact of critical illness and facilitate the process of rehabilitation and coping with the transition from critical illness to health. These are the key messages to apply to your practice in this chapter.

- The impact of critical illness can be far reaching, and the psychological needs of patients can hinder or enhance their recovery.
- Meeting the psychological needs of patients and families requires emotional care as well as physical care.
- The caring practices related to clinical compassion, competence, confidence, conscience, commitment and comportment can make a positive difference to patient and family experiences of critical illness.
- Nurses can develop their emotional intelligence to facilitate the management of the emotional labour of caring as well as improving their potential for personal and professional development.

Further reading

National Institute for Health and Clinical Excellence (NICE) (2009) *Rehabilitation after critical illness, NICE clinical guideline 83*. London: National Institute for Health and Clinical Excellence.

This clinical guideline highlights the long-term effects of critical illness and how it is important to assess and support the patient following their discharge from critical care in order to improve patient outcome.

Useful websites

www.healthtalkonline.org/Intensive_care/Intensive_care_Patients_experiences

This website provides text and video clips of patient and family experiences of critical care and gives a balanced view of people's memories and experiences.

www.ics.ac.uk/patients_relatives/patients_relatives_section

The Intensive Care Society (ICS) provides guidance and support channels for patients and their relatives during and following admission to intensive care. The site provides printable booklets for patients and families as well as guidance for all levels of staff in critical care.

Chapter 12
Conclusion
Lessons learned – an action plan for practice

Desiree Tait

The chapters in this book have provided an opportunity for you to explore the clinical assessment and rapid decision-making skills required to manage acute and critically ill patients. The patient case studies and scenarios used in the book are fictional, but the physiological and psychological data used have been based on real situations. This has provided each patient's story with an authentic thread as their stories began to unfold. By reading the scenarios and practising the activities in each chapter you have had opportunities to rehearse situations in a safe environment and reflect on their outcome. The key messages that have emerged from this book have been visited in each chapter and can be summarised as the following.

- Always use a comprehensive, systematic and holistic approach to nursing assessment.
- Always interpret the findings from your assessment and determine a diagnosis of the current situation.
- Always respond to your findings in a timely manner, ensuring that you communicate your concerns and review the situation.
- Always provide support and protection for vulnerable people in your care.
- Always provide a person-centred approach to care and ensure that you acknowledge and communicate the wishes and concerns of the patient and families when delivering nursing care.
- Always demonstrate a collaborative approach to care.

Within the chapters we have discussed the care of acutely ill patients and those at risk of deterioration in acute and critical care settings in both community and hospital environments. It is important to recognise that the rapid decision-making skills required to manage these patients safely are the same wherever the patient is located, although the access to interventions may vary depending on the facilities available. It is not the intention of the authors to provide you with the skills to become a critical care nurse but rather to show you how you can influence patients' care for the better and have a positive impact on their outcome in all clinical settings where patients are at risk.

Developing an action plan for practice

In your role as a senior student and as a qualified nurse your priority will be to ensure that you meet the standards and competencies set by the NMC (2010). After you qualify as a registered nurse, these standards will continue to be a basis from which to develop your practice as well as to teach others. According to Benner et al. (1999), rapid assessment and understanding of the patient's condition is based on the nurse's ability to interpret, recognise and respond to patterns and trends in the patient's behaviour and physiological data. This ability comes from knowledge and experience developed over time, the presence of leadership and organisational skills, and the presence of clinical forethought (the ability to anticipate and act on potential problems). The development towards proficient and expert practice involves the refinement of clinical knowledge and evidence-based practice so that an intuitive understanding of practice is achieved. In order to continue to develop and expand your clinical decision-making skills, we have identified five action points that you can use on the journey.

1. *Never lose your willingness to learn*: Nursing and health care practice is a dynamic and innovative environment; use every opportunity you have to learn and develop your practice.
2. *Know your patients and always be receptive to their condition*: The patient or client is the person who lives with the experience of their condition. They know and sense when something has changed and it is reasonable to assume that knowing and understanding your patient will help you to interpret their condition quickly and effectively.
3. *Reflect on your nursing experiences and question the issues raised*: When reflecting on your practice, question and challenge your decision making. Can you justify the decisions you made with an evidence base? How strong is that evidence base? Do you need to explore this issue in more detail?
4. *Combine your knowledge from experience with evidence-based practice*: Clinical reasoning and decision making can be guided by an evidence base such as clinical pathways and care bundles. It is also important to remember that each patient is an individual, and the clinical value of all evidence-based interventions needs to be judged in the context of individualised patient care.
5. *Continue to work collaboratively with colleagues and demonstrate emotional intelligence when communicating with others*: In order to collaborate effectively with others you need to be aware of your own emotions and their impact on others, know your strengths and limitations, and have a sense of self-worth. You need to have an empathic awareness of others, with political and social awareness, so that you can interpret and manage communication between individuals and groups.

These action points will guide you on the path to professional maturity when involved in direct care and when collaborating with others. Nursing is a dynamic and exciting profession with a continuing demand for questioning of and learning from practice and is a journey to be enjoyed.

Glossary

abrasive trauma   a process of wearing away a surface area of the skin/mucous membrane by friction resulting from trauma.

activated partial thromboplastin (APPT)   a measure of the efficiency of activation and duration of clotting time.

acute pain   pain that is temporary, resulting from surgery, an injury or an infection.

acute pancreatitis   a sudden and often severe inflammation and swelling of the pancreas. The pancreas is normally protected from the digestive enzymes that it produces; however, during an acute episode the pancreatic enzymes begin to digest the tissue of the pancreas. In severe cases this is described as acute necrotising pancreatitis. The most common cause is alcohol abuse.

adenosine triphosphate (ATP)   a chemical in cells that is able to release energy during a chemical reaction. It is the major source of energy for all the body's cellular functions.

aldosterone   a hormone that increases the reabsorption of sodium ions and water. This increases circulating blood volume and blood pressure.

aminophylline   a drug used to prevent and treat wheezing, breathlessness and dyspnoea associated with asthma and COPD. It works by relaxing and dilating the bronchi in the respiratory system and making it easier for the patient to breathe. Side effects include an increase in heart rate and risk of cardiac arhythmias, restlessness and irritability.

angiotensin converting enzyme (ACE)   an enzyme secreted by the pulmonary endothelial cells to act as a catalyst in the conversion of angiotensin I to angiotensin II.

angiotensin I   an inactive chemical that is triggered by the release of renin and activated by an enzyme to produce angiotensin II.

angiotensin II   once activated by the renin angiotensin system, angiotensin II exerts a vasoconstrictor effect, increases a sensation for thirst and ultimately increases blood pressure.

antidiuretic hormone (ADH)   a hormone that increases the concentration of urine (osmolarity) and reduces the excretion of water by the kidneys. It also has a powerful vasopressor effect, thus increasing peripheral resistance and blood pressure; also known as vasopressin.

benzodiazepines   a group of drugs that have a number of sedative, muscle relaxant and amnesic effects. They are prescribed to relieve anxiety, induce sleep, as an anticonvulsant in the management of seizures, to relieve muscle spasm and to manage alcohol withdrawal.

beta agonist   a group of drugs that include salbutamol and are effective in causing bronchodilation. They relieve bronchospasm, wheezing and breathlessness. They are most frequently administered by the inhalation route and can have an effect in just a few minutes. Side effects include an increase in heart rate and risk of cardiac arhythmias, restlessness, anxiety and shaking/tremor in the limbs. The side effects usually last for only a few minutes.

bradykinin   a protein found in the body that when released causes vasodilation during the inflammatory response and when systemic can lead to a reduction in blood pressure.

carbon monoxide poisoning   occurs following enough inhalation of carbon monoxide gas (CO), a colourless, odourless and tasteless toxic gas found in appliances such as gas boilers and in exhaust fumes from older vehicles. CO poisoning is potentially fatal because of the ability of the CO to bind to haemoglobin. As a result the body is unable to carry enough oxygen to the tissues and organs.

cardiogenic shock   occurs when there is an inadequate circulation of blood to the body's organs and tissues due to primary failure of the ventricles of the heart to function effectively.

central venous pressure   the blood pressure in the vena cava, the blood vessel returning to the right atrium of the heart. Measuring the CVP allows you to measure the amount of blood returning to the heart and is an indication of fluid balance in the circulation. When the CVP is low, the patient may be suffering from hypovolaemia; when it is high, the patient may be fluid overloaded or suffering from right-sided cardiac pump failure leading to a backlog of blood in the venous circulation.

cerebrospinal fluid   a bodily fluid that occupies the subarachnoid space and the ventricular system around and inside the brain and spinal cord.

chronic pain   pain that lasts longer than three months. It is different from acute pain in that it is not easy to find the cause, and diagnosis can reveal no injury in the body at all, yet the patient can be experiencing very debilitating pain.

Colles fracture   a fracture of the distal radius in the forearm with dorsal (posterior) displacement of the wrist and hand. The fracture is sometimes referred to as a 'dinner fork' or 'bayonet' deformity due to the shape of the resultant forearm.

compensatory stage of shock   the second stage of shock, which occurs when the body has triggered compensatory mechanisms to improve blood supply to organs and tissues in order to maintain homeostasis.

complement system   a system made up of plasma proteins that react with one another to make pathogens such as a bacterial infection easier to break down and digest. Overall the system induces a series of inflammatory responses that help to fight infection.

distributive shock   occurs when there is inadequate circulation of the blood to the body's organs and tissues due to the systemic dilation of blood vessels. This is found, for example, in anaphylactic shock and septic shock.

dobutamine   a drug that stimulates the beta receptors of the sympathetic nervous system. It is used to improve cardiac output in patients with cardiogenic shock.

dopamine   a neurotransmitter acting on receptors in the brain. It acts on the sympathetic nervous system to increase heart rate and blood pressure.

dyspnoea   a term used to describe difficult or laboured breathing and is often associated with breathlessness.

empirical antibiotic therapy   refers to the commencement of treatment before a firm diagnosis is reached. In the case of infection patients are prescribed broad spectrum antibiotics until the microorganisms are cultured and diagnosed. The antibiotics may then be changed if the microorganisms are not sensitive to the prescribed medication.

escharotomy   provides a release of tissue constriction that compromises the underlying structures, whether those are circulatory or respiratory structures. Untreated, the tissue constriction will lead to loss of limbs by compromising the circulation, or death by constricting chest movement and preventing lung expansion.

Guillain-Barré Syndrome   a neurological disorder that occurs when the body's immune system attacks part of the peripheral nervous system. This can lead to symptoms such as muscle weakness, paralysis, breathing difficulties and an unstable heart rate and blood pressure. Most people who get the disease can make a complete recovery although initially the disorder is considered a medical emergency.

haemoserous fluid   blood-stained fluid that is leaking from the wound (haemoserous means 'stained with blood').

histamine   chemical released by the mast cells as part of the inflammatory response. Its action is to dilate blood vessels and increase capillary permeability to white blood cells in order to fight the pathogens in infected tissues.

hyperlipidaemia   refers to raised blood levels of cholesterol. Raised levels of cholesterol, in combination with other risk factors, can increase the risk of stroke and/or heart disease

hypovolaemic shock   occurs when there is inadequate circulation of the blood to the body's organs and tissues due to loss of blood or body fluids.

inflammatory mediators   various chemicals that, when released by immune cells, cause vasodilation and bring about an inflammatory response.

initial stage of shock   the first stage of shock, which occurs when the body begins to recognise and respond to a reduction in blood flow to the organs and tissues.

inotropic therapy   includes the use of drugs that improve the force of muscle contraction and are said to have a positive inotropic effect.

interleukins   a family of proteins that control some aspects of the immune response. They do this by conveying signals between white blood cells.

intubated (intubation) the placement of a flexible, cuffed tube into the trachea in order to maintain an open airway and facilitate processes such as assisted ventilation, administering anaesthesia during surgical procedures and to prevent airway obstruction and/or accidental inhalation of toxic substances; referred to as tracheal intubation.

invasive ventilation intubation and respiratory support provided either to assist normal breathing or, in some cases, to replace normal breathing. Patients usually require sedation when receiving invasive ventilation.

iron lung a large cylindrical steel chamber. Patients laid in the chamber with only their head and neck free. The chamber was airtight, and at set intervals the atmospheric pressure inside the chamber was reduced to lower than atmospheric pressure. This change in pressure reduced the work of breathing for the patient and the patient was able to take a deeper breath (increase their tidal volume). When the interchamber pressure returned to normal, the patient exhaled normally.

kinins any of a group of substances formed in body tissue in response to injury.

laparoscopic cholecystectomy the surgical removal of the gall bladder using a minimally invasive technique.

leukotrienes any of a group of physiologically active substances that possibly function as mediators during acute inflammatory responses.

lymphocytes a family of white blood cells that are responsible for defending the body against infection and damage. They include B lymphocytes that attack bacteria and toxins, and T lymphocytes that attack cells that have been taken over by a damaging organism such as a virus or by cancerous cells.

mandibular refers to any tissue or bony structure that makes up the lower jaw.

midazolam a short-acting drug of the benzodiazepine family. It is used to induce sedation and amnesia before and during medical procedures, to treat acute seizures, and as sedation in the management of ventilated patients.

monocyte a type of white blood cell that plays a role in the inflammatory and immune response. Monocytes can develop either into dendritic cells that play a role in the antibody antigen response or into macrophages, which are cells that eat other damaged cells.

muscarinic antagonist a group of drugs, also known as anticholinergic drugs, and include Ipratropium bromide (Atrovent). They work causing bronchodilation in the lungs and are used to treat asthma and COPD. They are administered by inhalation and patients may complain of a dry mouth when taking these drugs.

nephrotoxic the poisonous effect of medication, on the kidneys.

neutrophil the most common type of white blood cell that acts as the first line of defence when the inflammatory response is triggered. Neutrophils will recognise anything that should not be present in the body as an invader and destroy it.

nitric oxide a compound that acts as a vasodilator, helps to regulate the uptake of oxygen in cells and can destroy viruses and cancer cells as part of the immune system.

nitrous oxide a colourless, non-flammable chemical compound used in medicine for its analgesic, anaesthetic and anxiolytic effects, usually administered by inhalation and distributed through the lungs by diffusion.

nociceptive pain is caused by stimulation of peripheral nerve fibres that respond only to stimuli approaching or exceeding harmful intensity, the most common categories being thermal, mechanical and chemical.

nociceptors sensory neurons that are found in any area of the body that can sense pain either externally or internally.

non-steroidal anti-inflammatory drugs (NSAIDs) a group of drugs that have analgesic, anti-inflammatory and antipyretic effects. These drugs can cause dyspepsia and gastric ulceration.

obstructive shock occurs when there is inadequate circulation of the blood to the body's organs and tissues due to physical obstruction of blood flow from the heart or aorta, such as in cardiac tamponade when the pericardial sac fills with blood and squashes the ventricles.

obstructive sleep apnoea a condition characterised by repeated intermittent obstruction or collapse of the upper airways during sleep, often accompanied by loud snoring. The patient experiences periods of apnoea (no breathing), tiredness and lethargy.

oedema an excessive accumulation of serous fluid in the intercellular spaces of tissue.

osmolarity   the measure of the concentration of solute particles in a solution.

phagocytosis   the process that cells such as neutrophils use to destroy dead or foreign cells by ingesting or engulfing them.

phlebitis   the inflammation of the walls of the vein.

pneumothorax   a collection of air that has leaked into the space between the layers of the lung sac. The lung is contained in two sacs: the visceral and parietal layers of the pleura. The parietal layer lines the thoracic wall and the visceral layer covers all the surfaces of the lungs. Leakage of air into the pleural space can build up and cause the lung to collapse. When this happens the patient is unable to take a deep breath and becomes breathless and dyspnoeic.

prednisilone   a type of corticosteroid. It has anti-inflammatory properties and is used to control inflammatory diseases such as asthma, COPD and rheumatoid arthritis. If a patient has been prescribed prednisilone for more than three weeks, it will have altered the body's normal steroid production and the drug will need to be reduced slowly to avoid a steroid crisis. Patients taking steroids also have reduced immunity and should carry a drug alert or treatment card with them at all times in case of a sudden emergency.

primary survey   a methodical process used to quickly identify immediate life-threatening injuries and conditions that require immediate attention.

progressive stage of shock   the third stage of shock, which occurs when the underlying cause of the shock has not been corrected and the body is no longer able to compensate for the reduction in blood flow. Cell damage becomes more severe over time and can be irreversible.

prostaglandins   a group of substances that influence a number of body functions such as the dilation and constriction of blood vessels, control of blood pressure and the inflammatory response. They are also influential in the promotion of uterine contractions during childbirth.

prothrombin time (PT)   a blood test that measures how long it takes blood to clot. It is also known as an INR test (international normalised ratio) when the results are standardised to facilitate wider standard interpretation.

pulmonary embolism   occurs when a blood vessel supplying blood to the lungs becomes clogged by a blood clot or embolus. This prevents an amount of blood from perfusing the alveoli and as a result the body receives a reduced supply of oxygenated blood.

refractory stage of shock   the fourth and final stage of shock, which occurs when the body's organs begin to fail due to a sustained lack of oxygen and nutrients; eventually the organs completely fail and this leads to death.

renin-angiotensin-aldosterone mechanism   a hormone system that helps to regulate fluid balance and blood pressure. The system forms part of the body's response to shock.

secondary survey   a complete examination of the patient from top to toe, both front and back.

septic shock   shock caused by decreased tissue perfusion and oxygen delivery as a result of severe infection and sepsis, and it can cause multiple organ dysfunction syndrome (formerly known as multiple organ failure).

somatic pain   pain arising from tissues such as skin, muscle, tendon, joint capsules, fasciae and bone.

tachypnoea   rapid breathing or respiration.

tissue necrosis factor (TNF)   one of the cytokines that are influential in the inflammatory response. TNF induces cell death in cancer cells and is involved in stimulating the inflammatory response.

vascular permeability   the degree to which one substance allows another substance to pass through it.

vasodilation   the widening of blood vessels resulting from the relaxation of the muscular wall of the blood vessels.

vasopressin   see antidiuretic hormone (ADH).

ventilation   a method used to assist spontaneous breathing. The techniques available include non-invasive ventilation where respiratory support is provided through a tight-fitting mask and the patient continues to breathe with support.

visceral pain   pain arising from the internal organs; patients state the pain feels like squeezing, cramping or pressure.

References

Adam, S, Odell, M and Welch, J (2010) *Rapid assessment of the acutely ill patient.* Oxford: Wiley Blackwell.

Aldemir, M, Ozen, S, Kara, O et al. (2001) Predisposing factors for delirium in the surgical intensive care unit. *Critical Care*, 5: 265–70.

American College of Surgeons (2008) ATLS, *Advanced Trauma Life Support program for doctors.* Chicago IL: American College of Surgeons.

American Psychiatric Association (2000) *Diagnostic and statistical manual of mental disorders*, 4th edition. Washington DC: American Psychiatric Association.

American Psychiatric Association (2004) *Practice guideline for the treatment of patients with acute stress disorder and posttraumatic stress disorder.* Arlington VA: American Psychiatric Association.

Arend, E and Christensen, M (2009) Delirium in the intensive care unit: a review. *Nursing in Critical Care* 14(3): 145–54.

Babaev, A, Frederick, P, Pasta, D, Every, N, Sichrovsky, T and Hochman, J for the NRMI Investigators (2005) Trends in management and outcome of patients with acute myocardial infarction complicated by cardiogenic shock. *Journal of the American Medical Association*, 294(4): 448–54.

Beard, H (2005) Does intermediate care minimise relocation stress for patients leaving the ICU? *Nursing in Critical Care*, 10(6): 272–78.

Beauvais, A, Brady, N, OShea, E and Quinn Griffin, M (2011) Emotional intelligence and nursing performance among nursing students. *Nurse Education Today*, 31: 396–401.

Beel-Bates, C and Rogers, A (1990) An exploratory study of sundown syndrome. *Journal of Neuroscience Nursing*, 22: 51–52.

Benner, P, Hooper-Kyriakidis, P and Stannard, D (1999) *Clinical wisdom and interventions in critical care.* Philadelphia PA: W B Saunders Company.

Bersten, A and Soni, N (eds) (2003) *Oh's intensive care manual*, 5th edition. Oxford: Butterworth Heinemann.

Bickley, L (2008) *Bates' guide to physical examination and history taking*, 10th edition. Philadelphia PA: Lippincott, Williams and Wilkins.

BMA (British Medical Association), Resuscitation Council (UK) and RCN (Royal College of Nursing) (2007) *Decisions relating to cardiopulmonary resuscitation.* London: British Medical Association.

Boe, J, Dennis, J H, O'Driscoll, B R, Bauer, T T, Carone, M, Dautzenberg, B, Diot, P, Heslop, K and Lannerfors, L (2001) European Respiratory Society guidelines on the use of nebulisers. *European Respiratory Journal*, 18: 228–42.

Bone, R, Balk, R, Cerra, F et al. (1992) Definitions for sepsis and organ failure, and guidelines for the use of innovative therapies in sepsis. *Chest*, 101: 1644–55.

Borthwick, M, Bourne, R, Craig, M et al. (2006) *Detection, prevention and treatment of delirium in critically ill patients.* United Kingdom Clinical Pharmacy Association. Accessed at: www.ics.ac.uk/intensive_care_professional/standards_and_guidelines/ukcpa_delirium_2006.

Boykin, A and Schoenhofer, S (1993) *Nursing as caring: a model for transforming practice.* New York: National League for Nursing.

Brainard, J and Deutschman, C (2010) What are the indications for intubation in the critically ill patient? In Deutschman, C and Neligan, P *Evidence based practice for critical care.* Philadelphia PA: Saunders Elsevier: 11–14.

Bray, K, Hill, K, Robson, W et al. (2004) British Association of Critical Care Nurses' position statement on the use of restraint in adult critical care units. *Nursing in Critical Care*, 9(5): 199–212.

Bridges, E and Dukes, S (2005) Cardiovascular aspects of septic shock: pathophysiology, monitoring and treatment. *Critical Care Nurse.* 25(2): 14–40.

BTS (British Thoracic Society) and SIGN (Scottish Intercollegiate Guidelines Network) (2009) *British guidelines on the management of asthma.* London: British Thoracic Society.

Carbery, C (2008) Basic concepts in mechanical ventilation. *Journal of Perioperative Practice*, 18(3): 106–14.

Carpenito, L (2000) *Nursing diagnosis: application to clinical practice*, 8th edition. Philadelphia PA: Lippincott.

Chaboyer, W, Kendall, E, Kendall, M and Foster, M (2005) Transfer out of intensive care: a qualitative exploration of patient and family perceptions. *Australian Critical Care*, 18(4): 138–45.

Cole, E (2009) *Trauma care: initial assessment and management in the Emergency Department*. Oxford: Blackwell Publishing.

Cook, P (2006) *Neurological workshop*. Manchester: Greater Manchester Strategic Health Authority.

Creed, F and Spiers, C (2010) *Care of the acutely ill adult: an essential guide for nurses*. Oxford: Oxford University Press.

Creed, F, Dawson, J and Looker, K (2010) Assessment tools and track and trigger systems, in Creed, F and Spiers, C (2010) *Care of the acutely ill adult: an essential guide for nurses*. Oxford: Oxford University Press.

Daniels, R (2011) Heart of England sepsis screening tool. Accessed at: www.survivingsepsis.org/Site CollectionDocuments/Sepsis%203+3%20tool%20ward%20_2_.pdf.

Daniels, R and Nutbeam, T (2009) *ABC of sepsis (ABC series)*. Oxford: Wiley-Blackwell.

Dayton, E and Henriksen, K (2007) Communication failure: basic components, contributing factors and the call for structure. *Joint Commission Journal on Quality and Patient Safety*, 33(1): 34–47.

de Wit, M, Wan, S Y, Gill, S, Jenvey, W, Best, A, Tomlinson, J and Weaver, M (2007) Prevalence and impact of alcohol and other drug use disorders on sedation and mechanical ventilation: a retrospective study. *Anaesthesiology*, 7(3): 1–9.

Department of Health (2000) *Comprehensive critical care: a review of adult critical care services*. Accessed at: www.dh.gov.uk/en/Publicationsandstatistics/Publications/PublicationsPolicyAndGuidance/DH_4006585.

Department of Health and NHS Modernisation Agency (2003) *The national outreach report 2003*. London: NHS Modernisation Agency.

Dougherty, L and Lister, S (2008) *The Royal Marsden Hospital manual of clinical nursing procedure*. 7th edition. Oxford: Wiley-Blackwell.

Duffield, C, Roche, M, Diers, D, Catling-Paull, C and Blay, N (2010) Staffing, skill mix and the model of care. *Journal of Clinical Nursing*, 19: 2242–51.

Dunlop, C and Whyte, P (2010) Is oxygen toxic? in Deutschman, C and Neligan, P (eds) *Evidence based practice for critical care*. Philadelphia PA: Saunders: 45–50.

Ely, E, Truman, B, Shintani, A, Thomason, J, Wheeler, A, Gordon, S, Francis, J, Speroff, T, Gautam, S, Margolin, R, Sessler, C, Dittus, R and Bernard, G (2003) Monitoring sedation status over time in ICU patients: reliability and validity of the Richmond Agitation-Sedation Scale (RASS). *Journal of the American Medical Association*, 289(22): 2983–91.

Ely, W and Vanderbilt University (2010) *Confusion assessment method for ICU (CAM-ICU): the complete training manual*. Nashville TN: Vanderbilt University.

Fairbrother, G, Jones, A and Rivas, K (2010) Changing model of nursing care from individual patient allocation to team nursing in the acute inpatient environment. *Contemporary Nurse*, 35(2): 202–20.

Finfgeld-Connet, D (2007) Meta synthesis of caring in nursing. *Journal of Clinical Nursing*, 17: 196–204.

Fleming, S and Todd, N (1998) Cardiorespiratory physiology, in Shuldham, C (1998) *Cardiorespiratory nursing*. London: Stanley-Thornes.

Franklin, C and Matthew, J (1994) Developing strategies to prevent in hospital cardiac arrest: analysing responses of physicians and nurses in the hours before the event. *Critical Care Medicine*, 22: 244–47.

Fulbrook, P and Mooney, S (2003) Care bundles in critical care: a practical approach to evidence based practice. *Nursing in Critical Care*, 8: 249–55.

Gao, H, McDonnell, A, Harrison, D A, Moore, T, Adam, S, Daly, K, Esmonde, L, Goldhill, D R, Parry, G J, Rashidian, A, Subbe, C P and Harvey, S (2007) Systematic review and evaluation of physiological track and trigger warning systems for identifying at-risk patients on the ward. *Intensive Care Medicine*, 33: 667–79.

Goleman, D. (1998) *Working with emotional intelligence*. London: Bloomsbury Publishing.

Gowda, R, Fox, J and Khan I (2008) Cardiogenic shock: basics and clinical considerations. *International Journal of Cardiology*, 123: 221–28.

Gray, J (1987) *The psychology of fear and stress*. Cambridge: Cambridge University Press.

Green, D, Ervine, E and White, S (2003) *Fundamentals of perioperative management*. London: Greenwich Medical Media.

Greenhalgh, J, Vanhanen, V and Kyngas, H (1998) Nurse caring behaviours. *Journal of Advanced Nursing*, 27(5): 927–32.

Grossbach, I, Chlan, L and Tracy, M (2011) Overview of mechanical ventilator support and management of patient- and ventilator-related responses. *Critical Care Nurse*, 31(3): 30–44.

Hall, J (2011) *Guyton and Hall: textbook of medical physiology*, 12th edition. Philadelphia PA: Saunders Elsevier.

Harrison, D, Welch, C and Eddleston, J (2006) The epidemiology of severe sepsis in England, Wales and Northern Ireland, 1996–2004: secondary analysis of a high quality clinical database, the ICNARC case mix programme database. *Critical Care*, 10(r42): 1–10.

Hastings, M (2009) *Clinical Skills Made Incredibly Easy*. Philadelphia PA: Lippincott Williams.

Helmy, A, Vizcaychip, M and Gupta, A K (2007) Traumatic brain injury: intensive care management. *British Journal of Anaesthesia*, 99(1): 32–34.

Henderson, A (2002) Emotional labour and nursing: an under-appreciated aspect of caring work. *Nursing Inquiry*, 8:130–38.

Herndon, D N (2007) *Total burn care*, 3rd edition. London: W B Saunders.

Higgs, J, Jones, M, Loftus, S and Christensen, N (2008) *Clinical reasoning in the health professions* (3rd edition). Oxford: Butterworth Heinemann.

Hochschild, A (1983) *The managed heart: commercialization of human feeling*. Berkeley CA: University of California Press.

Hockman, J, Sleeper, L, Webb, J, Dzavik, V, Buller, C, Aylward, P, Col, J and White, H (2006) Early revascularization and long term survival in cardiogenic shock complicating acute myocardial infarction. *Journal of the American Medical Association*, 295(21): 2511–15.

Hopkins, A (1994) The trauma nurse's role with families in crisis. *Critical Care Nurse*, April: 35–43.

ICS (Intensive Care Society) (2007) *Sedation guideline*. London: Intensive Care Society. Accessed at: www.ics.ac.uk/intensive_care_professional/standards_and_guidelines/sedation_guidelines_2007.

ICS (2009) *Levels of critical care for adult patients*. Accessed at: www.ics.ac.uk/intensive_care_professional/standards_and_guidelines/levels_of_critical_care_for_adult_patients.

ICSI (Institute for Clinical Systems Improvement) (2009) *Diagnosis and treatment of chest pain and acute coronary syndrome (ACS)*. Bloomington MN: ICSI.

Identifying Sepsis Early Group (2006) *Identifying sepsis early*. Edinburgh: University of Edinburgh.

IHI (Institute for Health Care Improvement) (2009) *Improvement map: patient care processes: pressure ulcer prevention*. Accessed at: www.ihi.org/offerings/initiatives/improvemaphospitals/Pages/default.aspx.

IHI (2011a) *Rapid response team data collection and SBAR communication* tool. Accessed at: www.ihi.org/knowledge/Pages/Tools/SBARToolkit.aspx (accessed on 14 June 2011).

IHI (2011b) *Implement the IHI central line bundle*. Accessed at: www.ihi.org/knowledge/Pages/Changes/ImplementtheCentralLineBundle.aspx.

International Sepsis Forum (2003) *Promoting a better understanding of sepsis*, 2nd edition. Land O'Lakes FL: International Sepsis Forum.

Jarvis, H (2006) Exploring the evidence base for the use of non-invasive ventilation. *British Journal of Nursing*, 15(14): 756–59.

Jeffries, D, Johnson, M and Griffiths, R (2010) A meta-study of the essentials of quality nursing documentation. *International Journal of Nursing Practice*, 16: 112–24.

Jevon, P (2008) Neurological assessment part 1 – assessing level of consciousness. *Nursing Times* 104(27): 26–27.

Jevon, P and Ewens, B (2007) *Monitoring the critically ill patient*, 2nd edition. Oxford: Blackwell Publishing.

Kapborg, I (2000) The nursing education programme in Lithuania: voices of student nurses. *Journal of Advanced Nursing*, 27(5): 927–32.

Kennedy, A (2009) Meningitis and encephalomyelitis, in Bersten, A and Soni, N *Oh's intensive care manual*, 6th edition. London: Butterworth-Heinemann: 47, 583–92.

Khademian, Z and Vizeshfar, F (2007) Student nurses' perceptions of the importance of caring behaviours. *Journal of Advanced Nursing*, 61(4): 456–62.

Kiekkas, P, Theodorakopoulou, G, Spyratos, F and Baltopoulos, G (2010) Psychological distress and delusional memories after critical care: a literature review. *International Nursing Review*, 57: 288–96.

Kinrade, T, Jackson, A and Tomnay, J (2009) The psychological needs of families during critical illness: a comparison of nurses' and family members' perspectives. *Australian Journal of Advanced Nursing*, 27(1): 82–8.

Kumar, P and Clark, M (2001) *Clinical medicine*, 4th edition. London: Saunders.

Lassen, H C A, Bjorneboe, M, Ibsen, B and Neukirch, F (1954) Treatment of tetanus with curarisation, general anaesthesia and intratracheal positive pressure ventilation. *Lancet*, ii: 1040–44.

Lawrence, P and Fulbrook, P (2011) The ventilator care bundle and its impact on ventilator-associated pneumonia: a review of the evidence. *Nursing in Critical Care*, 16(5): 222–34.

Levy, M, Fink, M, Marshall, J et al. (2003) International sepsis definitions conference. *Critical Care Medicine*, 31:1250–56.

Levy, M, Dellinger, R, Townsend, S et al. (2010) The surviving sepsis campaign: results of an international guideline-based performance improvement programme targeting severe sepsis. *Intensive Care Medicine*, 36: 222–31.

Lim, W S, Baudouin, S V, George, R C, Hill, A T, Jamieson, C, Le Jeune, I, Macfarlane, J T, Read, R C, Robert, H J, Levy, M C, Wani, M and Woodhead, M A (2009) Guidelines for the management of community acquired pneumonia in adults: Update 2009. Pneumonia guidelines Committee of the British Thoracic Society Standards of Care Committee, *Thorax* 64 (supp III).

Lynch M (2001) Pain as the fifth vital sign. *Journal of Intravenous Nursing*, 24(2): 85–94.

Mackintosh, C (2006) Caring: the socialisation of pre-registration student nurses: a longitudinal qualitative descriptive study. *International Journal of Nursing Studies*, 43(8), 935–62.

Martin, E A (ed.) (2010) *Oxford Concise Medical Dictionary*. Oxford: Oxford University Press.

Mattson Porth, C and Matfin, G (2009) *Pathophysiology: concepts of altered health status*, 8th edition. Philadelphia PA: Lippincott.

Mayer, J, Caruso, D and Salovey, P (1999) Emotional intelligence meets traditional standards for an intelligence. *Intelligence*, 27: 267–98.

McCaffery, M and Beebe, A (1993) *Pain: clinical manual for nursing practice*. Baltimore MD: V V Mosby Company.

McCaffery, M and Pasero, C (1999) *Pain: a clinical manual*. St Louis MO: Mosby.

McGloin, H, Adam, S and Singer, M (1999) Unexpected deaths and referrals to intensive care of patients on general wards. Are some cases potentially avoidable? *Journal of the Royal College of Physicians of London*, 33: 255–59.

McLuckie, A (2009) Shock – an overview, in Bersten, A, Soni, N and Oh, T E *Oh's Intensive Care Manual*, 6th edition. London: Butterworth-Heinemann: 97–104.

McQuillan, P, Pilkington, S, Allan, A, Taylor, B, Short, A, Morgan, G, Nielson, M, Barrett, D and Smith, G (1998) Confidential inquiry into quality of care before admission to intensive care. *British Medical Journal*, 316 (748): 1853–58.

Merritt, S (2009) Chronic obstructive pulmonary disease, in Smith, S A, Price, A M and Challiner, A (2009) *Ward based critical care: a guide for health professionals*. Keswick: M & K Publishing.

Migliozzi, J (2009) Shock, in Nair, M and Peate, I *Fundamentals of applied pathophysiology*. Chichester: Wiley-Blackwell: 86–100.

Mitchell, M, Courtney, M and Coyer, F (2003) Understanding uncertainty and minimising families' anxiety at the time of transfer from intensive care. *Nursing and Health Sciences*, 5: 207–17.

Molter, N (1979) Needs of relatives of critically ill patients: a descriptive study. *Heart and Lung – The Journal of Critical and Acute Care*, 8(2): 332–39.

National Clinical Guideline Centre (2010) *Delirium: diagnosis, prevention and management*. London: National Clinical Guideline Centre for Acute and Chronic Conditions.

NHS Wales (2010) *1000 lives plus: how to guide 6: rapid response to acute illness*. Accessed at: www.1000livesplus.wales.nhs.uk.

NICE (National Institute for Health and Clinical Excellence) (2007a) *Acutely ill patients in hospital: recognition of and response to acute illness in adults in hospital, NICE clinical guideline 50*. London: NICE.

NICE (2007b) *Head injury: triage, assessment, investigation and early management of head injury in infants, children and adults*. London: NICE.

NICE (2008) *Lipid modification, NICE clinical guideline 67*. London: NICE.

NICE (2009) *Rehabilitation after critical illness, NICE clinical guideline 83*. London: NICE.

NICE (2010a) *Delirium: diagnosis, prevention and management, NICE clinical guideline 103*. London: NICE.

NICE (2010b) *Quick reference guide to delirium: diagnosis, prevention and management, NICE clinical guideline 103*. London: NICE.

NICE (2010c) *Chronic obstructive pulmonary disease, NICE clinical guideline 101*. London: NICE.

NICE (2010d) *A review of acutely ill patients in hospital: recognition of and response to acute illness in adults in hospital, NICE clinical guideline 50*. London: NICE.

NICE (2011) *NICE Pathways*. Accessed at: http://pathways.nice.org.uk/ (accessed 14 June 2011).

Nightingale, F (1860) *Notes on nursing: what it is what it is not*. New York: Appleton and Company. Accessed at: http://digital.library.upenn.edu/women/nightingale/nursing/nursing.html#XIII (accessed on 25 April 2008).

NMC (Nursing and Midwifery Council) (2008) *Standards of conduct, performance and ethics*. London: NMC.

NMC (2010) *Standards for pre-registration nursing education*. London: NMC.

NPSA (National Patient Safety Agency) (2007a) *Recognising and responding appropriately to early signs of deterioration in hospitalised patients*. London: NPSA.

NPSA (2007b) *Safer care for the acutely ill patient: learning from serious incidents*. London: National Patient Safety Agency.

O'Connor, M, Bucknall, T and Manias, E (2008) A critical review of daily sedation interuption in the intensive care unit. *Journal of Clinical Nursing*, 18: 1239–49.

O'Connor, M, Bucknall, T and Manias, E (2010) International variations in outcomes from sedation protocol research: where are we at and where do we go from here? *Intensive and Critical Care Nursing*, 26(4): 189–95.

O'Driscoll, B R, Howard, L S and Davison, A G (2008) *Guidelines for emergency oxygen use in adult patients: executive summary*. London: British Thoracic Society; also in *Thorax*, 63 (Supplement VI): vi1-vi68.

Page, V (2008) *ICU delirium: why it matters*. Accessed at: www.icudelirium.co.uk/why-it-matters (accessed on 19 December 2011).

Patrozou, E and Opal, S (2010) What is inflammation? What is sepsis? What is MODS? in Deutschman, C and Neligan, P (2010) *Evidence based practice in critical care*, 24: 151–56.

Pattison, N (2005) Psychological implications of admission to critical care. *British Journal of Nursing*, 14(13): 708–14.

Porth, C M (1998) *Pathophysiology: concepts of altered health states*, 5th edition. Philadelphia PA: Lippincott-Raven.

Ramsay, M, Savego, T, Simpson, B and Goodwin, R (1974) Controlled sedation with alphaxolone-alphadolone. *British Medical Journal*, 2(920): 656–59.

RCP (Royal College of Physicians), BTS (British Thoracic Society) and ICS (Intensive Care Society) (2008) The use of non-invasive ventilation in the management of patients with chronic obstructive pulmonary disease admitted to hospital with acute type II respiratory failure. London: Royal College of Physicians. Accessed at: www.rcplondon.ac.uk/resources/non-invasive-ventilation-chronic-obstructive-pulmonary-disease.

RCP (2012) Policy responses and statements: NHS early warning score (NEWS). Accessed at: www.rcpe.ac.uk/policy/2011/nhs-early-warning-score.php.

Redden, M and Wotton, K (2002a) Third space shift in elderly patients undergoing gastrointestinal surgery: Part 1: Pathophysiological mechanisms. *Contemporary Nurse*, 12(3): 275–83.

Redden, M and Wotton, K (2002b) Third space shift in elderly patients undergoing gastrointestinal surgery: Part 2: Nursing assessment. *Contemporary Nurse*, 13(1): 50–60.

Resuscitation Council (UK) (2006a) (revised 2012) *Medical emergencies and resuscitation*. London: Resuscitation Council (UK).

Resuscitation Council (UK) (2006b) *Advanced life support*, 5th edition. London: Resuscitation Council (UK).

Riker, R, Fraser, G, Simmons, L and Wilkins, M (2001) Validating the sedation agitation scale with the bispectral index and visual analogue scale in adult ICU patients after cardiac surgery. *Intensive Care Medicine*, 27(5): 853–58.

Rivers, E, Nguyen, B, Havstad, S et al. (2001) Early goal directed therapy in the treatment of severe sepsis and septic shock. *New England Journal of Medicine*, 344: 699–709.

Roach, M. (1984) *Caring: the human mode of being, implications for nursing*. Toronto: Faculty of Nursing, University of Toronto.

Roach, M (2002) *Caring: the human mode of being: a blueprint for the health professions*, 2nd edition. Ottawa: CHA Press.

Royal College of Nursing (2003) *Defining nursing*. London: Royal College of Nursing. Accessed at: www.rcn.org.uk/_data/assets/pdf_file/0003/78564/001983.pdf.

Samuelson, K (2011) Unpleasant and pleasant memories of intensive care in adult mechanically ventilated patients: findings from 250 interviews. *Intensive and Critical Care Nursing*, 27: 76–84.

San Diego Patient Safety Council (2009) *Tool Kit: ICU sedation guidelines of care*. San Diego: San Diego Patient safety Council. Accessed at: www.chpso.org/meds/sedation.pdf.

Saunderson-Cohen, S (2002) *Trauma nursing secrets*. Philadelphia PA: Hanley & Belfus.

Schoenhofer, S (2001) A framework for caring in a technologically dependent nursing practice environment, in Locin, R (ed.) *Advancing technology, caring and nursing*. Westport CT: Auburn House: 1, 3–11.

Scott, C (2003) *Setting safe nurse staffing levels: RCN research report*. London: Royal College of Nursing.

Scottish Intercollegiate Guidelines Network (2010) *Management of chronic venous leg ulcers: national clinical guideline 120*. Edinburgh: Scottish Intercollegiate Guidelines Network.

Skaer, T L (1998) Cancer pain management. *American Journal of Pharmaceutical Education* 62: 182–89.

Smith, J (2005) Caring for multicultural patients: emotional intelligence as a framework for providing reflective health care. *International Journal of Health Care*, 9(2): 80.

Smith, J (2009) How to keep score of acuity and dependency. *Nursing Management* 16(8):14–19.

Smith, M and Segal, J (2011) Post-traumatic stress disorder (PTSD): symptoms, treatment and self help. Accessed at: http://helpguide.org/mental/post_traumatic_stress_disorder_symptoms_treatment.htm.

Smith, S A, Price, A M and Challiner, A (2009) *Ward based critical care: a guide for health professionals*. Keswick: M & K Publishing.

SSC (Surviving Sepsis Campaign) (2011) in Dellinger, R, Mitchell, M, Levy, M et al. (2008) Surviving sepsis campaign: international guidelines for management of severe sepsis and septic shock: 2008. *Intensive Care Medicine* 34(1): 17–60. Updated amendments accessed at: www.survivingsepsis.org/guidelines/.

Stayt, L (2009) Death, empathy and self preservation: the emotional labour of caring for families of the critically ill in adult intensive care. *Journal of Clinical Nursing*, 18: 1267–75.

Tait, D (2009) *A Gadamerian hermeneutic study of nurses' experiences of recognising and managing patients with clinical deterioration and critical illness in a NHS Trust in Wales*. Unpublished doctoral thesis: University of Wales Swansea.

Thompson, C and Dowding, D (2002) *Clinical decision making and judgement in nursing*. Edinburgh: Churchill Livingstone.

Tourangeau, A, Cranley, L and Jeffs, L (2006) Impact of nursing on hospital patient mortality: a focused review and related policy implications. *Quality Safe Health Care*, 15(4): 4–8.

Walsh, T and Ezz-El Din Saleh (2006) Anaemia during critical illness. *British Journal of Anaesthesia*, 97(3): 278–91.

Watson, R (2008) Research into ageing and older people. *Journal of Nursing Management*, 16: 99–104.

Wheeldon, A (2009) The respiratory system and associated disorders, in Muralitharan, N and Peate, I (2009) *Fundamentals of applied pathophysiology: an essential guide for student nurses*. Chichester: Wiley-Blackwell.

WHO (World Health Organisation) (1996) *Cancer pain relief*. 2nd edition. Geneva: World Health Organisation.

Williams, T, Martin, S, Thomas, L, Leen, T, Tamaliunas, S, Lee, K and Dobb, G (2008) Duration of mechanical ventilation in an adult intensive care unit after introduction of sedation and pain scales. *American Journal of Critical Care*, 17(4): 349–56.

Wilson, B (2007) Nurses' knowledge of pain. *Journal of Clinical Nursing*, 16(6): 1012–20.

Woodrow, P (2012) *Intensive care nursing: a framework for practice*, 3rd edition. London: Routledge.

Woodward, S and Waterhouse, C (2009) *Oxford Handbook of Neuroscience Nursing*. Oxford: Oxford University Press.

Zwarenstein, M, Goldman, J and Reeves, S (2009) *Interprofessional collaboration: effects of practice based interventions on professional practice and health care outcomes (review)*. London: John Wiley and Sons. Accessed at: http://onlinelibrary.wiley.com/doi/10.1002/14651858.CD000072.pub2/pdf/standard.

Index